D0398370

MAKE
AMERICA
HEALTHY
AGAIN

MAKE AMERICA HEALTHY AGAIN

How Bad Behavior and
Big Government Caused
a Trillion-Dollar Crisis

NICOLE SAPHIER, MD

BROADSIDE BOOKS
An Imprint of HarperCollins*Publishers*

This book contains information relating to health care. It should be used to supplement rather than replace the advice of your doctor or another trained health professional. If you know or suspect that you have a health problem, it is recommended that you seek your physician's advice before embarking on any medical program or treatment. All efforts have been made to ensure the accuracy of the information contained in this book as of the date of publication. The publisher and the author disclaim liability for any adverse effects arising from the use or application of the information contained herein.

HarperCollins books may be purchased for educational, business, or sales promotional use. For information, please email the Special Markets Department at SPsales @harpercollins.com.

FIRST EDITION

Library of Congress Cataloging-in-Publication Data has been applied for.

ISBN 978-0-06-296100-6

20 21 22 23 24 LSC 10 9 8 7 6 5 4 3 2 1

For Nicholas Anthony, whose mere existence
has been my greatest motivator.

For Hudson and Harrison, for insisting I play board games and
read bedtime stories, despite delaying work on this book.

For Paul, who stands beside me every day, and
lifts me up when I need a boost.

You cannot subsidize irresponsibility and expect people to become more responsible.

—THOMAS SOWELL

CONTENTS

INTRODUCTION

America, we are in a crisis.

This is not about an existential or political crisis or an economic or religious tumult. We are in the midst of an absolute, head-on, health care crisis.

I admit it's an unusual kind of crisis. In the past few years, research and ingenuity have yielded more advancements in the field of medicine than the decade before them. And that decade saw the rise of more technological wonders and advanced treatments than the century before it. In fact, by New Year's Day 2000, the average life expectancy in the United States had almost doubled from what it had been on New Year's Day 1900, rising from approximately forty-seven years to seventy-seven. It is wonderful that we were able to defy the laws of physics and safely send a man to the moon and back. But to double our lifespan in such a short period implies that we are on to something even greater: defying our own mortality.

As a physician, I witness firsthand every day how modern medicine has an impact on the lives of everyday people. However, the example closest to my heart is my own Uncle Joe.

He was a normal kid born to a normal family and grew up to be a normal man with normal kids and normal grandkids. That was not always the case for someone diagnosed with type 1 diabetes. Uncle Joe depended on a daily regimen of finger sticks and injections of insulin, a necessary hormone his own body deprived him of and without which he would have suffered a horrendous, early death. While that may not sound remarkable, consider the fact that had he been born just a few years earlier, this medicine would not have been available when he was a kid. He would likely not have survived to graduate college, let alone have his first son.

They say in life that timing is everything, and for Uncle Joe, this expression could not have been more spot-on. For while he was able to live into adulthood and raise his boys, years of battling diabetes caught up with his body, as it does with so many other of its victims. His kidneys failed, and he was again dying. This time, no medicine in the world would save him. What did save him, though, was a complicated surgical procedure in which he received a transplanted kidney and pancreas, the organ responsible for making the body's own natural insulin. After surgery, his kidney functioned at full strength, and his own body was making enough insulin so that he no longer needed to take the daily injections. Had his kidneys failed a decade before, he may have gone on daily dialysis with an average life expectancy of only a few years, and he would never have seen his first grandson.

Being born in the right year and suffering a condition at the right time allowed Uncle Joe to receive medical therapy that allowed him not only to live but to thrive. When his transplanted kidney began to fail—as often happens after a decade of extended life—he was again fortunate. He underwent a successful repeat kidney transplant, possible only by the advanced surgical technique, and even more revolutionary genetic sequencing technology identifying his own son as a 100 percent ideal match.

Uncle Joe was the lucky recipient of a breakthrough medicine that replaced his own body's missing insulin, a revolutionary surgery transplanting a functional kidney and pancreas, allowing him to survive a horrible demise from a crippled organ, and ultimately genomic sequencing pushed his life expectancy beyond another decade. All of these mortality-defying therapies had not been available the decade prior. He was always there at the right time.

However, at the same time that we've made so much progress, our costs have also been growing.

Each presidential administration during my lifetime and many before trumpeted that we are on the verge of a disaster. On October 10, 1952, President Dwight Eisenhower gave a speech in Salt Lake City in which he reiterated his opposition to socialized medicine while also recognizing that all Americans deserve basic medical care and that the system needed reform.

However, it wasn't until July 10, 1969, that President Richard Nixon proclaimed, "We face a massive crisis in this area. Without prompt administrative and legislative action, we will have a breakdown in our medical care system." This was considered the first time an administration declared such an emergency and it not only was a pivotal moment for health care but also marked the first attempt at a comprehensive health care reform.

Ronald Reagan, a hero of so many present-day Republicans, was even willing to raise taxes to expand the government program Medicare. "While I am opposed to socialized medicine, I have always felt that medical care should be available to those who cannot otherwise afford it." Although eager to recover from a difficult midterm election in 1982, Reagan's Medicare expansion might have been too generous for the nation's own good, causing continued rises in taxes and allotments for Medicare and Medicaid.

As the costs continued to soar, health care was further discussed by Barack Obama when he addressed Congress in 2009. "Our collective failure to meet this challenge—year after year, decade after decade—has led us to a breaking point." The latest report from the Centers for Medicare and Medicaid Services (CMS), published recently in *Health Affairs*, estimates national health expenditures will reach 20 percent of the gross domestic product (GDP) by 2027, and it included a series of colorful charts demonstrating theories on how and why costs have risen. The *New York Times*, the *Wall Street Journal*, and even the *New York Post* were quick to pick up on this headline and used even more flair to highlight that America is going bankrupt and that our health system is to blame for it. The problem is that the report and various media outlets failed to note an important point regarding their latest "catastrophic" projections: We are not in an immediate crisis, rather we are nearing our fifth decade of a growing problem.

It would be easy to think that innovation has driven these increased costs. However, pharmaceutical and medical device costs account for approximately 4 percent of the increased health care cost each year. The cost to develop and produce these novel discoveries is only one of the drivers of the rise in costs.

Health care in the United States now resembles a business venture and, like all successful business ventures, to function it must acquire administrative staff, legal counselors, information and technology specialists, marketing personnel, and an abundance of ancillary staff. This organizational compound, while good for overseers, adds on remarkable nonmedical expenses to the total cost of care, thus increasing health care spending. Therefore, it is not surprising that the highest-paid entities in health care today are not physicians, but corporate executives and high-level administrators.

Health care commercial greed is best reflected when evaluating the acquisition of drug rights, which is separate from the research and development of pharmaceuticals. There are numerous medications that small start-up companies buy the marketing rights to, and then increase the price for profit. These small companies do not have the burden of significant R&D debt as the original company did upon inventing the drugs. To recover the cost of acquiring the drug's rights and to make revenue, the small companies will increase the cost of the acquired medication. Sometimes the price rise is subtle over a period, but other times the price is increased abruptly, leaving many patients unable to afford the medication and facing the choice of having to forgo treatment.

Take the case of EpiPen® (epinephrine), a lifesaving medicine used to treat severe allergic reactions. Mylan Pharmaceuticals, Inc., purchased the product's marketing rights from Merck in 2007. At the time of sale EpiPen® cost approximately $57 and its annual sales were $200 million; today the same drug costs roughly $415 for a pack of two EpiPens,® with a short lifespan of one year until it needs to be replaced. The annual sale of this lifesaving drug today is more than $1 billion.[1] Did I mention the 2018 reported total income for the Merck CEO was $20,934,504?[2]

This is only one example of corporate greed taking with giving little in return. This obvious materialism regarding a single life-saving medication raises questions about moral ethics and fair practice regarding drug acquisitions and pricing in general. But the greed is not limited to the pharmaceutical companies; the hospital administrators are reaping the same seven- or eight-digit compensation packages. Consider this: the CEO for General Electric, a Fortune 500 company with about 300,000 employees, earned roughly $21 million in 2018. Interestingly, Jim Skogsbergh of Advocate Aurora Health, which has 70,000 employees, made $11.7 million in 2017—up by 42 percent from the previous year.

In the health insurance industry, the discrepancy is even more marked: Aetna CEO Mark Bertolini made $18.7 million in total compensation in 2016. I would be remiss if I didn't point out that the average salary of a general physician ranges from $150,000 to $180,000, despite spending three to four more years in educational training than the administrative staff dictating their every move. Physicians also often work longer hours.

Although there is a common criticism that health insurance companies and hospitals pay their CEOs too much, that's more reflective of the fact that CEO salary growth, on average, has far outpaced overall wage growth over the past several decades. So, while a seven- or eight-figure CEO salary seems absurd to most of us, it's in line with the corporate norm. And while US doctors are paid slightly more than their counterparts in other parts of the world, our physicians are highly skilled professionals who save lives, working long hours while saddled with the exorbitant cost of student debt after years of education.

In a free-market economy like that of the United States, it is assumed that when demand for a product increases, resources grow. This phenomenon often leads to an increase in supply, and the price of the product stabilizes and may even lower from market competition. But the reverse is true in the drug and insurance industry today; as the demand increases or remains stable, the industry keeps increasing the price regardless and the CEOs' salaries rise accordingly. Ultimately, all these increases are passed on to the consumer and the payer (the government or the private insurers).

However, as unreasonable as these salaries may seem, major establishments and highly compensated CEOs are necessary to manage the massive complex health systems. Such mammoth organizations have formed as small business medical practices have been run out of business by the Affordable Care Act, and large consolidations take over the health system.

Most physicians, hospitals, and even health insurers run on less than a 4 percent profit margin. Medical instrument and drug companies reap a larger margin of roughly 10 to 20 percent. However, it is their inventions, which exist independently of acquisition drug price hikes, that push us forward as a leading nation in health care advancement. Although politicians and grassroots organizations love to demonize these companies, and while fine-tuning with some oversight will improve the process, their portion of health care charges are nowhere near what "we the people" are costing us.

Here is the puzzle we are facing. Costs are rising, but we can't blame it all on R&D or profits or bureaucracy. In fact, we can't even say it's worth it as long as we are all living longer. We are not.

For the first time since 1993, the average US life expectancy dropped in 2015. Then again in 2016. And once again in 2017. It is not the older generations who are experiencing shortened survival. People in the United States are dying earlier. The frightening reality is that all of the prior medical marvels notwithstanding, our society is falling critically ill. We are losing too many Americans too early, and that is a monumental crisis we have yet encountered with all of our medical marvels. While historians may accurately point to world wars and pandemics causing major dips in populations, this downward spiral is an intrinsic part of our society's fabric. This is not a result of genocide or contagion; this is a result of numerous factors that pervade our society and afflict us like a plague. Some are the result of individuals' lifestyles; some are caused by deficient social integration. Many are caused by a system that is broken.

There are innumerable reasons we are in this crisis, and while some of the causes may be complex, there is one straightforward answer: If we do not rise to meet the challenge of this crisis, then America the Sick will ultimately be taken off life support.

Life expectancy gives us a snapshot of our overall health, and these sobering facts are telling us that we are losing too many Americans, too early, and too often, pointing us toward a crisis.

For me, the most important point that can be made is that a "health care crisis" itself is a nebulous phrase. Each legislative cycle echoes similar rhetoric to bring perceived calamity and urgency to a situation for political advantage. For most people, health care is personal because all people at some point find themselves in a vulnerable place where they depend on it. It's an excellent political tactic: Vote for me, and I will fix this *crisis* and save your life.

The fastest way to lower our costs, or at least to slow the upward trajectory, is to reduce the number of Americans who are sick.

According to the CDC, preventable chronic diseases account for 75 percent of our nation's health care spending. American health care costs as much as it does, in large part, because we have driven up the costs. The critical concentration should therefore be on how we live our lives and the preventative measures we can take to avoid costly illness.

So we have choices, America. We can continue to bankrupt our nation and pay more as we continue to lead the world in preventable illness. We can lose our rank as a global innovator by halting invention. Or we can get to the crux of the issue and rein in our poor lifestyles that have left our health system a thin veil of the personalized care we once knew.

We have come a long way on taming the complications of the body, but not very far in taming the complications of the mind.

Make America Healthy Again is a book about what happens when a huge swath of society decides their health is someone else's problem. Over the course of this book, we're going to look at the opioid epidemic, diabetes, doctor burnout, and the trillion dollars we spend on cancer every year. Through these stories, I will explain twin problems that have stirred our health care crisis.

The first is the inaccurate picture we have of the nation's health from TV and magazines. We consistently think our obstacles are different from what they actually are. We see diet books on the bestseller lists and celebrities looking younger and fitter in every photo. We misinterpret this to think the whole nation is eating kale and carrying a yoga mat around. We are healthy and looking for ways to get healthier. Nothing could be further from the truth.

Instead, the source of our greatest strength—medical innovation—has become our greatest weakness. We are looking to experts to solve our problems with pills and superfoods and surgeries. As a nation, we are getting unhealthier and hoping doctors will save us. This has negative repercussions across all of our society. We continue to make that mistake at our own peril.

The second, deeper issue is that the plan to fix this has made it worse. We have never been more responsible—and irresponsible—for our own outcomes. We don't exercise when we should or eat like we know we should eat. We don't take our pills, but we take our own lives. It's hard to comprehend how a health care system that promises to fix our problems, no matter what happens, will give people the incentive to do better.

There is certainly a valid argument in favor of removing profit as a motive from American health care. Advocates of a single-payer system commonly preach that health care is fundamentally different from other industries and, therefore, should not be profit-driven. However, opponents for a socialized health system contend that profit is essential for encouraging innovation and quality improvements. Either way, policy isn't plaguing America—we are.

The president and Congress must base any future health policies on reforms that will make America a healthier nation. Grandstanding from speculative leaders and politicians about the false accomplishments of policy are futile, as cost-containment policies have inadvertent consequences for us all. The power to regain functional control of our health system is not gone; it is time to refocus on how we can individually and collectively be less sick.

MAKE
AMERICA
HEALTHY
AGAIN

Chapter 1

THE AMERICAN HEALTH CRISIS

Health insurance is an invention of the twentieth century. In the early 1900s the average American spent about five dollars a year on health care, or roughly $131 today. Who needs insurance when your medical costs are minuscule?

Yet here's what health care in the nineteenth and early twentieth centuries looked like: Americans tried to fix real ailments with fake potions that amounted to little more than snake and lavender oil. Hospitals even operated inside courthouses during times of war, where soldiers and indigents essentially went to die. Medical care may have been cheap, but it was also medieval. It wasn't exactly a system built for saving lives.

Death is a universal reality, but the conditions or diseases that cause death have changed over time. In the early 1900s Americans were primarily dying from influenza, tuberculosis, and diarrheal diseases such as cholera. In 1918 millions of people around the globe died from the Spanish flu epidemic. As time went on, leading causes of death continued to be communicable diseases like measles, cholera, and other common respiratory or gastrointestinal (GI) tract viruses. Many perished at young ages from illnesses for which there was little or no treatment.

Times have changed. Our technology has advanced rapidly, enabling us to develop treatments (and, in many cases, cures) so that we in the United States no longer succumb to the same infectious disease pandemics that afflicted previous generations. Today, very few people are dying from infectious diseases for which we have no known cure. We have even overcome the more recent AIDS epidemic, caused by the human immunodeficiency virus (HIV), with marked advances in prevention and treatment specific to this virus. Did anyone think in the 1980s that within a short time we would have a medication that has a nearly 100 percent prevention rate for HIV? If you did, bravo. Personally, I never would have guessed.

By the mid-1900s, with far fewer cases of communicable diseases thanks to the advent of vaccinations and antibiotics, the emerging leading causes of death were heart disease, cancer, and unintentional injuries (motor vehicle accidents, overdoses). From the late 1950s through the early 1990s, while cancer and heart disease incidence went untouched, the death rate from accidents decreased. This reduction coincided with implementation of a 55-mph speed limit during the first energy crisis in the 1970s and the mandated use of seat belts in most states beginning in 1984.

Our increased longevity is one of the greatest medical achievements of the modern era. On average, Americans today can expect to live nearly thirty years longer than did our predecessors living at the turn of the twentieth century.

Between 1880 and 1945, US life expectancy rose from 40 to 65 years thanks to greater understanding of hygiene, improvements in sanitation and clean water supply, and the discovery of most antibiotics and vaccines. Americans could see not only their children but their grandchildren grow up and enjoy their time in retirement.

What is interesting and disheartening, however, is that we seem to have hit a standstill. Today, after seventy years of innovation, heart disease and cancer are still the top two causes of death in the United States.

Even more alarming is the fact that, on some fronts, Americans' health is growing worse. The United States has just witnessed a fall in life expectancy for the third year in a row—from a high of 78.9 years in 2014 to 78.6 years in 2017. The three-year drop represents the longest multiyear decline in life expectancy since the years 1915 to 1918, when the decrease was mostly attributable to World War I and the devastating 1918 influenza pandemic. As we approach a century of battling the same two top causes of death, why haven't we made any progress on these? Or have we?

The significant decrease in communicable-disease death rates combined with the high birth rates that followed World War II resulted in the vast baby boom generation. The first baby boomers reached retirement age in 2011, and we are now witnessing the abundant health needs of a large, aging population. While improved detection and treatment of chronic diseases have resulted in an overall declining mortality trend, those improvements have also increased the percentage of treated disease in the population. That in turn has resulted in an overall increase in the number of people living with chronic illness and consequent health care expenditure.

Today, instead of vast numbers of immediate deaths from plague and war, a new and rather unsettling era of sickness is tormenting our nation: self-inflicted chronic diseases. Given our access to top-level medical care in this country, how is it possible that, even as Americans are living longer, they are living with more illness? The answer lies in us as individuals and in our society collectively.

As medical advancements continue to improve health, and more baby boomers enter their retirement years, the demand for medical services is growing. Thus, spending on health care is rising along with these trends by an order of magnitude.

Increased Longevity Has Given Us Greater Responsibility for Our Own Health

In September 2009 President Barack Obama delivered an address to Congress on health care. In it he stressed that medical spending and insurance premiums were rising out of control: "We spend one and a half times more per person on health care than any other country, but we aren't any healthier for it. This is one of the reasons that insurance premiums have gone up three times faster than wages. It's why so many employers—especially small businesses—are forcing their employees to pay more for insurance, or are dropping their coverage entirely." Noting that the "health care system is placing an unsustainable burden on taxpayers," the president stated: "Put simply, our health care problem is our deficit problem."[1]

So, how did the cost of the American health system spiral into a $22 trillion deficit? A budget deficit is not necessarily a crisis in itself, despite what many believe. In fact, it can even increase economic growth by placing money in the pockets of businesses and families, thereby in theory creating a stronger economy. However, there is a tipping point with deficits, and as our health care costs are continuing to climb and we are not benefiting from a healthier America, that scale will begin to tip out of our favor. It may already have done so.

Prior to World War II, in the era when influenza and other infectious diseases claimed the most lives, the majority of Americans paid for their own medical care, either directly to their chosen doctor or through prepayment plans offered to certain groups of workers. Blue Cross nonprofit health insurance was created in 1929 to offer teachers guaranteed hospital care in return for a fixed monthly fee. Similar Blue Shield plans covered physician services.

Back then, health insurance was in fact insurance: the insured person prepaid a set amount to cover hospitalizations and surgeries that would not have been affordable if paid for out-of-pocket.

As World War II came to an end, the US government was determined not to repeat the economic devastation Germany faced after World War I. Following the war, Germany attempted to recover by way of increased social spending. Germany started creating transportation projects and modernizing energy in an effort to combat the rising unemployment rate. Yet the returns from income taxes were not enough to stave off the devastation of war. Social spending continued to rise at an unbelievable rate while the country was faced with foreign reparation payments they could not afford. Thus, Germany began printing vast amounts of money, sending the country into a state of super-inflation and economical collapse.

Intent on not falling in the same cyclical trap, Presidents Truman and Roosevelt decided to avoid social spending by granting political concession to labor without violating wage and price controls in a time of desolation. The federal government exempted employer-paid health insurance benefits, allowing off-the-books raises for employees in the form of nontaxable health benefits.

This unreported compensation in the form of health insurance benefits created an enormous tax advantage for employer-sponsored group health insurance plans over smaller individual policies, under which incidental medical expenses were purchased by employees with their own after-tax dollars. Additionally, under the group plans, employers received 100 percent of employees' federal, state, and city tax deductions for the cost of health benefits. Thus, a foundation was laid in the American health insurance industry for employer-sponsored group plans. This model functioned quite well while medical costs were low and employees stayed with the same company for their entire career. However, when medical costs began to rise, and employees started changing jobs more often, the system began to show signs of stress.

In response to the rising costs of group benefits, employers started restricting coverage, increasing the employee's cost to participate, and even cutting out health insurance benefits entirely. Not only did the out-of-pocket cash responsibility for the employee increase, but the cost of monthly premiums did as well. Perhaps if the insurance premiums had not risen, the out-of-pocket costs would have been more palatable since cash payments for medical expenses were not a new concept. In fact, in 1970 roughly 40 percent of personal health expenditures were self-pay; with low insurance costs, this was considered acceptable. Yet, since 2008, average family premiums have increased at a rapid pace—twice as fast as the rise in workers' earnings and three times as fast as inflation.[2]

An interesting article in the *New York Times* in May 2018 blamed our exponential rise in health care costs on a lack of regulation: "Other countries have been able to put limits on health-related prices and spending. The United States has relied more on market forces, which have been less effective."[3] It is true that American health spending has pulled away from that of other countries over recent decades. This is due in large part to an expansion of government-funded programs like Medicare and Medicaid without holding down prices, including the cost of technology adoption, as other countries do.

In today's horror stories about surprise medical bills, as reported by journalists such as Steven Brill and Sarah Kliff, medical treatments are followed by bankruptcy and despair. Such stories provide examples of overinflated expenses on hospital invoices without a thorough explanation of the causes underlying the rise in costs. For instance, an article by Kliff in *Vox* highlights a pricing issue:

Look at the price of a common antibiotic ointment called
bacitracin (you might know it better by its brand name,
Neosporin). The bills in our database show that one hospital
in Tennessee charged a patient a pretty reasonable $1 for
bacitracin—while another hospital in Seattle charged $76 for
the exact same ointment. Since prices aren't made public, it was
impossible for these (or any) patients to know whether they were at
a hospital that charges $1 for a squirt of antibiotic ointment or one
that charges 76 times that amount.[4]

Here is the missing piece to such stories: The bloated prices on most medical invoices are not the prices the patient or even the insurer would ever pay. Moreover, while the Defense Department was recently embarrassed about paying $10,000 for toilet seat covers for military planes, Medicare and Medicaid payment rules mean that the government pays even less than a private payer would for the services listed on medical invoices. Thus hospitals and physicians exaggerate prices because they are rarely paid what they charge, whether by the private insurer or a government plan. They are paid a percentage of their billed charges; therefore prices are inflated to ensure adequate compensation for services rendered. And often, when patients receive bills from the hospital or specialty doctor who provided urgent care, it is because the insurance company has refused to pay.

The real pièce de résistance missing in the article is the fact that an ailment requiring an over-the-counter antibiotic ointment is often easily and cheaply remedied at the local drugstore. However, if the patient went to the emergency department for that ailment, as in the cases described by the authors, is the hospital wrong to charge for the time and resources expended to treat a non-urgent issue? This is a contentious question. Put differently, while the evidence may show that high prices charged by doctors and hospitals are a major reason why medical costs account for a large and grow-ing share of the nation's GDP, those prices are not at the monu-mental level that many media outlets would have you believe. In fact, while prices may be increasing, the demand for services has risen at a higher rate. While inflated prices and system inefficien-cies explain part of the rising costs of health care, they don't ex-plain away the needlessly high demand for such care. Health care becomes costlier when a population ages and people live longer. Therefore, it's not surprising that half of the increase in spending comes from increased utilization of services.

For most people, rising insurance premiums are at the center of the health care debate. As government programs like Medicare, Medicaid, and the Patient Protection and Affordable Care Act (usually referred to as the ACA, or Obamacare) have led to more people having access to coverage, there has been an increased overall demand for medical services—resulting in higher costs. In addition, increases in the incidence of chronic conditions like diabetes and heart disease have had a major impact on price in-creases: the two diseases alone are responsible for 85 percent of medical costs and affect nearly half of all Americans.

Here's the bad news: Americans are slowly recognizing the harsh but unavoidable reality that (1) the *quality* of our extended lives is becoming increasingly compromised because of poor stew-ardship of our health, and that (2) the attendant increase in health care expenditures results in decreased financial security.

As America's fiscal health declines, individual health crises, such as heart disease, cancer, and mental illness, are causing mil-lions of workers reaching retirement age to experience shorter and less active retirements than their parents enjoyed. In other words, our increased life expectancy hasn't translated into more time enjoying life, more time with family, or more time living health-ily. Along with the problems besetting the country's aging baby boomers, younger populations (especially those between 24 and 44) are confronting a rising death rate.

I'm sure it will shock nobody to hear that Americans eat too much, drink too much, and are sedentary for far too many hours a day. In terms of our eating habits, if you travel to Europe you'll notice a striking difference between people on the streets of Paris or Milan and Americans, the most obvious being our waistlines. In European restaurants and markets, you'll also notice less processed food and sugary beverages.

A study by the World Health Organization estimates that 80 percent of cases of cardiovascular disease, including heart attacks and strokes, could be prevented if Americans would stop using tobacco, eat a healthier diet, and exercise more. Likewise, 40 percent of cancer cases may be prevented by the same three changes.

We don't make the necessary lifestyle changes partly because we have come to expect our system to pick up the pieces of our bad choices, and there is little motivation to do otherwise. As a result, even though we have access to the best medical technology and lead the world in advanced education, entrepreneurship, and technological innovation, we are faring the worst in terms of obesity, metabolic syndrome, and cardiovascular disease. (I hope nobody throws us a parade for achieving that distinction.) So what do we have to show for our financial investments in our health system? Why isn't a healthier life one of them? Three reasons: We don't trust our doctors, we want to blame other people for our problems, and we like instant gratification.

We Don't Trust Our Doctors

In an age when information we disagree with is considered "fake news," regardless of its source or validity, it should come as no surprise that this concept has spread beyond politics. The term "fake news" is commonly used to delineate fabricated media stories but is also being applied to broader subjects. With the inception of the internet and every social media platform, all health and wellness articles, largely non-factual, are widely accessible to people. This helps explain why younger generations have little respect for physicians and devalue their expert medical opinions.

The health crisis in this country has spread into almost every corner of American society, and there is plenty of blame to go around. The culmination of the rising cost of medical care coupled with the growing prevalence of sickness is plaguing our nation. Medical professionals themselves have played a role in diminishing trust: not only are physicians finding themselves increasingly pressured to prescribe medications but, with increasing government oversight, they also have less time to spend with patients, which undermines the chances of building a meaningful relationship. Nobody likes to talk about this, but the increased number of people abusing opioids is a direct result of big business and government putting themselves in the examining rooms across the nation and enforcing their own agendas. Doctors now spend as much time making sure boxes are checked so they are compensated for their work as they do speaking to their patients. The patient has morphed into an ancillary person in the room because the real relationship is between the insurance payer (private or public) and the doctor. So why would we expect anything other than a lack of patient trust when doctors are barely looking them in the eye? This loss of confidence translates to Americans no longer relying on experts for guidance. Instead, the internet has become the expert in all matters, and the physician is merely the avenue to get the treatment for the search engine "diagnosis." A doctor's education and experience are disregarded in exchange for Dr. Google, because if it's on the internet it must be right. Right?

We're reaping exactly what we sow—both in the doctor's office and outside of it. We have succeeded in bringing monumental advancements in health services to Americans while concurrently we have allowed increased bureaucratic intrusion into the system. All the while, individuals are not held accountable for their contributions to the overuse of such services. As the country undergoes the financial consequences, we have the audacity to complain about it.

We Want to Blame Others for Our Problems

If you switch the station from reality TV to the top news outlets, you'll see how invested we are in the narrative of social responsibility, whether politically, economically, or environmentally. Where is our parallel obligation to a person's *individual* responsibility to their health?

We blame fast-food chains and soda makers for our nation's obesity rates—sometimes even slapping taxes on the products to deter people from consuming them—but at some point we must stop placing the blame and burden on others and acknowledge that it's our own choosing to consume these products that is causing our sickness as a nation. In fact, a survey by the National Center for Health Statistics of the Centers for Disease Control and Prevention (CDC) indicated that, from 2013 to 2016, nearly 40 percent of Americans said they had eaten fast food on a given day.[5]

The wellness industry may be booming in popularity, and large numbers of Americans may *say* they are eating healthier, but facts don't lie. CDC data show that 90 percent of adults are not consuming the federal government's recommended daily amounts of fruits and vegetables, despite their claims of opting for healthier food.[6] We don't need a report to tell us that. We only need to go to any public place and look around, and we can see for ourselves that obesity rates are continuing to increase across America. So, if people are claiming to be leading healthier lives, what is going wrong? As people tend to cast blame elsewhere, we blame our unhealthy diet on the industry that produces our favorite foods and makes them far too convenient and accessible for us to resist. It's not our fault that we can't fit into our jeans—it's their fault.

McDonald's says its restaurants sell approximately 75 hamburgers per second. In the United States, you will never travel more than 110 miles without seeing the famous golden arches, the symbol that reminds you of the deliciousness that waits inside.

We are all looking for a means to lessen the chaos of daily life and steal a few minutes while juggling various responsibilities. During the workweek, we find ourselves constantly in search of the perfect work/life balance (whatever that is). Often we feel there isn't time to prepare healthy meals at home or to sit down in a "slow food" restaurant. When you decide to eat fast food, you save time by forgoing the dreaded grocery store runs, kitchen preparation, and cleanup. When you order fast food to take out, you don't even need to use a plate, a knife, or even a fork—you just eat with your hands out of the wrappers and then toss them out.

During working hours the battle is no different. Many of us have dedicated lunch hours, but unless we bring a nutritious meal we prepared ahead of time, we may opt for the efficiency and convenience of fast food; it may even be our only option. Not only does the food tempt us with high salt and sugar content, but given how cheap and convenient it is, it's no wonder four in ten Americans consume fast food on a daily basis.

So, we have blamed the fast-food industry for the temptation of its products, and we want to point the finger at the chains for our health problems. Let's be honest, eating healthy takes time and effort—and even if it didn't, we don't want to give up our greasy fries for broccoli.

In recent years, activists and organizations called on McDonald's to offer healthy options to its customers. There has also been legislation requiring chain restaurants to provide calorie counts and/or nutritional information on the food they serve. Here's the deal, though: McDonald's *is* a fast-food burger place—is it really their obligation to provide *anyone* with a healthy option? It's your right to walk into—or out of—any restaurant you choose, but it's not your right to demand they serve what you want. McDonald's takes in over $20 billion from their 14,000 US-based locations annually ($24.6 billion worldwide). Although McDonald's did cave under pressure to decrease the marketing of their less healthy offerings, if Americans actually stopped providing multimillion-dollar revenues to companies that don't solely serve healthy food, then they might actually revamp their entire menu to regain those lost earnings.

In 2004, McDonald's received negative publicity thanks to the documentary *Super Size Me*, by the independent American filmmaker Morgan Spurlock. In the film, Spurlock documented a thirty-day period in which he ate only McDonald's food. The film presented the negative health effects not only on his physical appearance but on his psychological well-being. It also delved into the national influence of the fast-food industry, including how it encourages a less nutritious diet for its own profit. Following the release of the film, McDonald's eliminated the "super-size" option on its menu and introduced healthier menu items. Although the company denied it did so because of the movie, clearly, McDonald's changed because of free-market pressures—it wanted to maintain market share.

Here is the harsh reality, though. Even with the new healthier choices added to the menu, McDonald's french fries (340 calories for medium) and Big Mac (563 calories) remain the top two ordered items.

The recommended daily calorie intake depends on various factors, like your sex, height, weight, and physical activity level. You need more calories when you're pregnant, highly active, or looking to gain weight, and fewer calories if you're sedentary or trying to lose weight. For the average adult, however, the long-time recommendation has been about 2,000 calories per day for women and 2,500 for men. Yet Americans eat an average of 3,600 calories per day. If people consume a Big Mac plus french fries, approaching 1,000 calories, for one meal, it's not hard to see how they exceed the recommended daily calorie count. On average, Americans weigh more than people from any other country in the world. We may demand wellness options, yet as a nation, we still lead the world in obesity.

This trend has been going on for quite some time. Our medical marvels continue to advance, and our treatments keep us alive longer, but it is our indulgent behavior that is now costing our nation more.

As a physician, I am growing increasingly frustrated and overwhelmed by the extent of administrative invasion into the realm of medicine to rein in the rising costs of health care. I don't think it is reasonable that many Americans are pushed into a subpar system because individuals aren't being held accountable for their lifestyle decisions—especially since it is exactly these decisions that are resulting in drastic exploitation of our system and the subsequent rising expenses. I appreciate that my property taxes help offset the costs of public education, road repair, and law enforcement, because that's how society works—and some levels of health care are no different. Yet when it comes to altering my professional environment and my family's access to quality medical care to cope with costs from other people's self-induced disease, my patience wears thin.

Will it take restructuring the entire system before we take responsibility for our health? The national conversation is trending toward single-payer health care as a dramatic solution. But I don't want a nationalized health system. As someone who leads a healthy lifestyle, I shouldn't be forced to bear the brunt of the pressures placed on the system by my cigarette-smoking, obese neighbors. Neither should you.

We Want Instant Gratification

On one hand, our demand for better health care results has spurred innovation, placing the American health system among the world's most advanced. On the other, our need for immediate results has led to an inflated sense of entitlement. People don't want to work for their health, they want innovation to make a simple cure. Instant gratification reigns supreme in America.

There's no better embodiment of this cultural phenomenon than reality television. Our version of royalty is the family who defines reality TV: the Kardashians. The Kardashian family members are champions and symbols of the new rage of image alteration, exemplifying the notion that you can look however you want to look with minimum effort and a wad of cash. While cosmetic procedures have existed for decades, they are experiencing a new surge in popularity. There were 17.7 million cosmetic procedures performed in 2018, according to the American Society of Plastic Surgeons.[7] As the Kardashians have shown, a person's appearance can be significantly altered by a variety of cosmetic procedures, including surgery, as well as hair extensions, makeup contouring, and then further airbrushing of your image.

Rather than working out, spending money on legitimate health needs, and consuming more nutritious foods, we are demanding the instant indulgence that plastic surgery, fad diets, and photo filters give us. That way we can look like we, too, deserve to be a social-media celebrity. We used to enjoy designer purses, designer watches, and designer dresses. Now, we are demanding designer bodies.

I'm seeing people's impatience with the work involved in wellness and their desire for personal transformation shaping their health care expectations, too. The patience to wait even two weeks for an appointment to see a physician for a non-urgent matter is running short. Over time, we'll see more walk-up health clinics in local drugstores, where you can be seen by a nurse promptly, because you have decided you can't wait to see the expert physician. Let's be clear: the medical cases for which you go to the store clinic aren't so dire that you have to be seen *urgently*, because people can't actually be treated at those sites for anything other than mild illnesses. Anything alarming and you will be sent to the emergency room. Why is it that Americans are willing to sacrifice medical knowledge for instant attention? By doing so, we are inadvertently pushing ourselves toward a complete government takeover of our health care system.

Fewer doctors are available, and some are considered too expensive. Instead of improving our system to increase access to physicians across the country, we are rationing out personnel to triage patients. This is a glimpse of what is to come if we implement a single-payer system before addressing the increased demands placed on our present system by preventable disease and impatience.

Look at our neighbor to the north, Canada, as an example of what can happen under a single-payer structure. The average wait time to see a specialty doctor (such as an orthopedic surgeon or a neurosurgeon) in Canada is thirty-five weeks. Not three to five weeks, thirty-five. Likewise, in some provinces it can take up to a year to get an MRI. The average wait times in the United States? Three to six weeks to see a specialist, and just a few days for an MRI. By American standards, that's still not fast enough. Just look at the online patient satisfaction reviews. Despite drastically shorter wait times in the United States than in nearly every other country, Americans' biggest complaints are about wait times and the amount of time spent face-to-face with doctors.

Canada's publicly funded system provides preventative care and medical treatment by primary-care physicians along with access to hospitals and other medical services. Contrary to popular belief, it does not cover dental, ambulance, or vision, and only some prescriptions. For individuals who require these services, they will typically need to purchase a separate private plan.

On average, middle-class Canadians pay more than Americans in federal taxes. Canadians also cope with higher sales taxes and higher costs for imported goods to offset the costs of the health system. However, Canadians enjoy health insurance coverage without any out-of-pocket expenses (except their higher tax rates and all the services not covered under their insurance). However, the removal of cost sharing (co-pays, deductibles) is one reason that wait times for appointments are substantially longer in Canada than in the United States. Publicly funded health systems must continually balance the desire for prompt quality-of-life treatment with the need to deliver universal health care in a fair and impartial manner. (People who can afford a separate comprehensive private plan get priority appointments because they can afford it.) Rather than increasing the number of professionals or facilities to reduce the subsequent long wait times, the government insists on keeping costs low because it has to. So, the government accepts delayed care as a reasonable consequence of providing single-payer coverage.

Public-policy think tanks have often reported that roughly

50,000 Canadians receive nonemergency medical treatment in the United States and other countries every year because the health services in Canada lack the capacity to provide the universal care they promise.

What many Americans don't realize is that a system like Canada's discriminates against people in the middle and lower classes. Those without disposable income solely use the government-issued plans, but the wealthy pay the premium for private insurance. Guess who has longer wait times: government-insured individuals or the privately insured? The answer, of course, is those with only government insurance, who just so happen to be members of the middle and lower classes. It's like air travel: economy class seems okay until you have experienced the convenience of flying first class. To continue the analogy, flying private would be equivalent to the high-level concierge doctor that many well-known celebrities employ.

In the United States, people are increasingly calling for "Medicare for All"—but the same people don't recognize that a single-payer system intentionally rations care, and that means even slower access than we are accustomed to and which we already complain about. There is nothing worse for instant-gratification seekers than waiting, no matter how briefly—unless of course you are in the top 1 percent of our nation's wealthiest. The wealthiest Americans will not feel the hit of single-payer if adopted in the United States because they will pay a premium for high-level concierge health care while the rest of us shuffle along on the wait lists.

If the government "pays" for everything, every facet of the system suffers. How can anyone demand a single-payer system while also expecting instant gratification?

In November 2018, Supreme Court Justice Ruth Bader Ginsburg (often called RBG) suffered a fall and broke two ribs. During the medical evaluation of the injuries, two lung nodules were detected on her CT scan. Radiologists call these "incidentalomas," that is, a finding incidental to the reason the exam was ordered. At the end of January 2019, it was publicly announced that RBG had undergone surgery to remove early-stage lung cancers at one of the world's top cancer hospitals, Memorial Sloan Kettering Cancer Center in New York City.

Based on my professional experience, I can surmise that a radiologist interpreted RBG's initial CT scan and then communicated that interpretation to the ordering doctor (in typical cases, that might be an ER doctor or primary-care doctor). That doctor then had to relay the news to RBG and refer her to a specialist. She then likely had a consultation appointment with a lung specialist. Additional imaging, blood tests, and maybe even a biopsy were performed. Surgery was scheduled, preceded by a presurgical testing appointment. The surgery was performed, and she was discharged home. Typically, such a patient would return to work following at least two or three postsurgical follow-up appointments and maybe even physical therapy.

In RBG's case, from cancer detection to diagnosis to treatment to recovery, it was all accomplished in under three months: her fall occurred in November 2018 and she returned to the High Court in early February 2019. It is hard to know for certain how much time elapsed between the CT scan and surgery because we don't know the date of the CT scan. What we do know is that only a month elapsed between her fall and the completed surgery. How can anyone not marvel at that efficiency or the fact that a geriatric patient made such a remarkable recovery? Take away the Supreme Court justice part of this patient experience, the average time between cancer diagnosis and treatment initiation in the United States is in fact only twenty-seven days.[8]

Only seven months after her amazing recovery from the life-saving lung-cancer surgery, RBG announced that she had also completed radiation treatment for a pancreatic neoplasm during this time. Decades ago she underwent an invasive surgery for a pancreatic cancer, so it's difficult to discern if this was a recurrence or a new cancer. Although nearly impossible to guess her exact course without knowing the details, even the earliest stage of pancreatic cancer requiring radiation carries a 14–55 percent five-year survival rate with treatment; radiation treatments range anywhere from $15,000 to $100,000. We can say without a doubt that RBG, at the age of eighty-six, with four cancer diagnoses (colon, pancreas, lung, pancreas) in her lifetime, is a survivor and a very expensive one.

Naturally, any cancer diagnosis produces anxiety, and the fact that patients don't want to wait to begin treatment is understandable. Respect for a patient's sense of urgency is one reason why the United States leads the world in cancer treatment and outcomes. And rightly so! Urgent matters should be prioritized in our health care system. It's when we demand instant attention for nonessential medical problems that we go wrong. Our system can't continue to be quick and affordable if we continue to use it for flippant reasons.

What if RBG had fallen in Canada? Senator Bernie Sanders loves telling Americans that we need to emulate the Canadian single-payer system, so let's take a look at it. Again, there are many unknown variables that would determine the outcome, especially since RBG likely would have been air-evacuated to the United States for immediate attention, but let's pretend that wasn't an option or that she was anyone other than the Notorious RBG. Less than 15 percent of Canadian rural emergency departments have a CT scanner; in 2019, Canadians waited an average of thirty-two days for CT scans unless they had alarming symptoms indicating a serious diagnosis, such as a punctured lung or a damaged heart. Focal pain suspected of being a rib fracture after a fall would not have necessitated an immediate CT scan, if one was ordered at all. When a nonemergent CT scan is ordered in Canada, the radiologist sends the results to the ordering physician within a week, further delaying the process of getting results to the patient. Imagine if RBG hadn't had the CT scan at all because the pain from her broken ribs subsided after the month-long wait or she was in a location with no access to one? Her incidentaloma may never have been found, resulting in a later, more advanced lung-cancer diagnosis associated with a lower survival rate, requiring more severe treatments, and at a much higher financial cost.

In the Canadian system, patients are given "priority" rankings. When a doctor suspects that a patient has cancer, the patient can be ranked as priority 4, for which the protocol is to have the patient see a surgeon within 35 days of an appointment request. Once surgery has been decided on, the surgery is to be performed within 84 days of that decision—an egregiously long wait time. Thankfully, the average wait time for Canadian patients is considerably shorter, at 39 days, with 92 percent of patients undergoing cancer surgery within 49 days. So, based on very rough estimates, RBG would have waited roughly 30 days for her CT scan, 7 days for the results, and another 40 days or so for her surgery, putting the total wait time at approximately two and a half months, at best.

Admittedly, the time to surgery in a low-grade, early-stage lung cancer does not change prognosis much from one to two months. In the United States, robust screening programs allow us to detect more cancers earlier when they are easier to treat (I should also note here that Canadian cancer-screening regimens are a skeleton of what we have in the United States). Had RBG's cancer been a more aggressive form, the tumor might have doubled in size and/or spread outside of the lungs while she waited for surgery, greatly reducing her chance of survival.

Canada isn't an anomaly. Every nation that offers government-funded, universal coverage features longer wait times than in the United States. Under the National Health Service (NHS), the universal health care system in the United Kingdom, after the initial suspicion of cancer, 78.2 percent of patients start treatment within two months (62 days) of being *urgently* referred by their primary-care doctor. Urgent referrals are only for symptoms of an advanced cancer, not a smaller, earlier-stage one.[9]

Long wait times for medically necessary treatment are not just an inconvenience. They can, and do, have serious consequences such as increased pain and mental anguish, and they can also result in poorer medical outcomes—transforming potentially reversible illnesses or injuries into chronic, irreversible conditions, or even permanent disabilities, with possible loss of earnings because of the inability to work.

If the United States adopted a single-payer system, do we really think Americans would put up with longer wait times for treatment of serious illness? For treating minor ailments, do we really think our desire for instant gratification would just go away? More importantly, how would we continue to provide exemplary care? Given America's worsening health as a result of self-inflicted conditions and illnesses, can you imagine the economic debacle that would result under single-payer?

If you think health care in the United States is expensive and inaccessible now, just wait until it's "free." When the government makes medical care "free," consumers' demand for services will surge. Patients will have no incentive to limit their doctor visits or choose more cost-efficient providers. This ultimately results in longer wait times for everyone.

Although many Americans view the co-pay as a kind of punishment, they should realize it functions as a deterrent for running to the doctor for minor complaints. Under government-funded insurance, when patients are no longer paying a portion of the cost, we'll start seeing an uptick in minor ailments bringing people to doctors' offices and emergency departments. Increased visits will mean longer wait times and bump up the taxpayers' costs even further. When we are faced with a two-month wait to get a doctor's appointment, we will have no one to blame but ourselves.

A Country of Victims or Achievers?

When people succeed, we congratulate the individual. When people make a mistake or fail, on the other hand, we're inclined to make excuses for them, or to blame society. Why are we reluctant to call out individuals for their own bad performance or decisions that have negatively affected them?

Look at self-made men like Andrew Carnegie and Kenneth Langone. Carnegie was born in a tiny cottage in Scotland in 1835, the son of a handloom weaver who moved his family to America in 1848. Carnegie, began working while still a boy, worked his way up in the railroad industry, made profitable investments, and in the 1870s founded a steel company that revolutionized the American steel industry. In retirement, having become one of the richest people in late-nineteenth-century America, he focused on philanthropy. Langone, a noted investor and philanthropist worth billions, was born in 1935 to an Italian American working-class family on New York's Long Island. He worked multiple jobs while completing his education. Langone then headed to Wall Street, where with smarts and hard work he climbed the ladder of success.

High-achieving men like Carnegie and Langone didn't use their humble beginnings as an excuse not to aim for success. Instead, they worked arduously to become the best in their fields and acquired a fortune in the process. Today, many Americans seem more inclined to make excuses for failure than to try harder to succeed. In fact, many seem content to view themselves as victims, not taking responsibility for their own problems.

When did our great nation turn into a country of victims?

We have become a coddled society, and it's evident in our medical system. Just one example is that doctors have become reluctant to tell people they are overweight out of fear of being accused of shaming their patients. Yes, there are many things in life that we can't control, including genetics and environmental factors that predispose us to many medical conditions. But we do have control over many other factors to reduce those risks or eliminate the chance of certain diseases altogether. Individuals can become healthier by making sound choices and following through on them.

Our health outcomes are largely predicated on our behavioral choices, not necessarily which doctor we go to or which insurance company we choose. If you find excuses to make bad choices in hopes that your doctor or socialized medicine will help you, then you'll be seriously disappointed. Physicians aren't miracle workers; we can only work with what we're given.

In fact, that's all any of us can do: make the best of our circumstances.

A New National Dialogue

We live in a great nation, but we're currently dealing with turmoil in the health care industry, in the political arena, in our schools, and in neighborhoods hit by the opioid crisis. Daily I hear people expressing discontent with one or another aspect of life in America.

The truth is, our behaviors are what got us here in the first place. On an individual basis, the behaviors that make you discontented in America will make you equally unhappy and unhealthy in Canada or Europe.

The ideas in this book won't always be easy pills to swallow (pardon the pun), but they are based on the proud heritage of the American founding. America was created on the principle that people are born with certain rights—life, liberty, and the pursuit of happiness—to be protected by a government of the people. Our forefathers envisioned a society grounded in individual responsibility. In that spirit, I have written this book as a first step toward opening a larger national dialogue about the state of America's health crisis.

How to Read This Book

I have read far too many self-help books, opinion essays, and scientific articles trying to break down the minutiae of various diseases and how to fix each one. That's not what this book is about.

I'm not here to preach the exact steps we should follow to be healthy, because I am far from a wellness expert. Nor is this a book pushing a partisan political agenda, because whether you are right, left, or center, no health policy will be successful in our country without Americans' taking control of their individual health.

My goal is to reframe your thinking, so we can bring to light not only how our individual behaviors are affecting our personal outcomes but how they're negatively affecting the entire health care system.

The days of paternalistic medicine are over. Patients are no longer expected to blindly follow doctors' orders without asking questions and thinking things through for themselves. You are the quarterback of your health care team. The ultimate capacity for good judgment lies with you. As a physician, I am here to give you information, interpret it for you, and give you options, but ultimately the decision to act is up to each of us, individually.

As Americans, we enjoy freedom and personal choice. I'm sharing my knowledge with you in this book to help you make the right choices for yourself.

Who Am I?

The life I'm leading could have turned out very differently. Not only did I grow up in a divorced, blended household, but I also faced a life-altering decision at a young age, when I became pregnant during my senior year of high school. I had to ask myself if I would be a victim of my circumstance or if I would forge ahead to continue following my dreams of becoming a physician.

So here I am. Once a single teenage mother, I am now married with three children. I'm a board-certified, nationally known radiologist at Memorial Sloan Kettering Cancer Center, America's top cancer center. In addition to my advocacy for legislative initiatives at the national and state levels, I hold a seat on a Centers for Disease Control and Prevention advisory committee, am a contracted contributor for Fox News Channel, and have been a featured medical and health policy expert on other major networks, including Fox Business Network, MSNBC, ABC, and HLN.

As I have spoken to a wide array of politicians, medical experts, and patients over the years, I have developed a new passion for examining and responding to our country's attitude about health care. I want people to take a more nuanced view of the situation facing America and see the system for what it is: a complex but solvable problem.

I'm far from perfect. I certainly don't exercise every day, I love chocolate, I drink wine, and my kids use their iPads more than anyone would recommend. I'm not vegan, and I don't do keto. But I think my professional experience as a physician gives me a good perspective on some of the problems plaguing our country.

America is sick, and the blame doesn't rest solely on Big Pharma's profit mongering, our country's socioeconomic disparities, government intrusion, or doctors' overprescribing tendencies. No—we are all to blame. It's our obligation to take a good hard look in the mirror and face up to what we're doing to add to the health crisis in this country.

This book will serve as your mirror.

Chapter 2

WHY IS HEALTH CARE
SO EXPENSIVE?

The American Medical Association (AMA), a national association of physicians, was founded in 1847. In the twentieth century, led in large part by the AMA, organized medicine became an important force for change. Medical professionals joined together to establish standards of medical practice, such as clean hospitals, sound pharmacological research, and well-educated and -trained doctors. Patients began to expect medicine to uphold these standards and no longer blindly accepted their fate. Although these were important steps forward, the concept of *preventive medicine* was not yet known. In some ways, we still haven't fully acknowledged the reach of diseases we can prevent, despite being inundated with wellness tips everywhere we look.

Fast-forward to the 1960s. In the first half of the twentieth century, national health care expenses had consistently increased. President John F. Kennedy introduced legislation to develop a taxpayer-funded plan for the aged, who were most afflicted by illness. JFK faced significant pushback by legislators who feared the beginnings of socialized medicine, and his bill did not pass. After Kennedy's assassination in 1963, Lyndon B. Johnson assumed the presidency and picked up where Kennedy left off. In 1965 he signed the bill that laid the groundwork for our present-day Medicare and Medicaid systems. Designed to help the elderly, disabled, poor, and mothers who had to stay home, these systems were meant to cover medical costs for people who were unable to gain coverage through an employer-sponsored plan.

Our vulnerable populations were taken care of. What went wrong for the rest of the population?

Shifting Expenses

Medicare and Medicaid started as noble endeavors, but they've become plagued with a host of problems.

When Medicare was first implemented, the average life expectancy was under 70. Now, Americans on average are living to nearly 79. As a result, people are receiving Medicare benefits for a significantly longer period than when the program started. Despite the increase in life expectancy, there has been no adjustment of the minimum age at which you can start receiving Medicare benefits.

When someone runs out of Medicare funds or they need long-term care, they have to use Medicaid to cover costs they can't pay on their own. If you're admitted into a nursing home, for example, Medicare doesn't pay for it—Medicaid does. Moreover, people used to go to nursing homes when they were near death, so this allotment was small. Now, people are living in nursing homes for years, sometimes ten or more, requiring hundreds of thousands of dollars' worth of care.

Who's paying for that? The taxpayer. In other words, we all are. Of course we want to care for our elderly and vulnerable, but as their longevity costs more, so do the treatments they are receiving.

It's one thing to subsidize costs for those who cannot afford it. Every American should receive medical treatment when in need.

That is what government assistance was created for. It's a completely different scenario when there are people on Medicaid or Medicare who are otherwise capable of obtaining employer-sponsored coverage. Also, some of those who receive government coverage are making poor decisions—smoking, drinking excessive amounts of alcohol, eating a poor diet, not exercising—that harm their health and increase the cost of their government-funded care.

Very little has been done to reduce the costs of health care in the United States, which is both more expensive than ever and an alarmingly big chunk of GDP. In 1960 health care spending was about 5 percent of US GDP. In 2017, it totaled $3.5 trillion, accounting for 17.9 percent of GDP.[1] That's an enormous increase. It would be nice to say that high prices are just a necessary side effect of our technologically advanced medical system, but the reality is that prices also reflect exploitation of the system.

How Did We Get Here?

Identifying a pattern leading to elevating prices is helpful to a certain extent, but teasing out the reasons behind it is another matter. Yes, drug prices are too high, hospital stays are too expensive, and the cost of maintaining electronic medical records is too high (thank you, Affordable Care Act). But none of those individual problems provides the complete picture. The root of the spending epidemic is much more complex and a system-wide problem.

Health-services payout is projected to continue growing faster than our GDP, up to 19.9 percent by 2025. This is an unsustainable path. Even my kindergartner could draw a line chart to see this isn't going to end well for our nation.

Prices rise when demand increases. With so many people demanding treatment for nonessential and essential care alike, we're seeing the prices rise to coincide with that demand.

Oppressive regulation doesn't solely drive prices down; rather it drives down quality and access. In fact, regulation may actually increase prices because of the administrative burden it can place on a system. As a physician, I'm in a profession that is aggressively overseen by powerful regulatory boards from the hospital itself, private medical associations, and the government. Simply maintaining those regulatory standards is exhausting, not to mention expensive. In addition, I'm taxed, I pay licensing fees, I pay malpractice insurance, and I pay all sorts of allowances that further drive up the overhead costs of being a doctor.

Likewise, a hidden rivalry between physicians and hospitals does nothing to alleviate the problem of costs. You see, as a consumer you have options: if you want to go to hospital A one week and hospital B the next week, you are able to. However, in an age of connectivity, it is often the case that those two hospitals will fail to communicate with each other regarding what treatments you've received. This lack of communication results in duplicate diagnostic tests and treatments, all of which are billed for. Your life literally depends on accurate and efficient communication among health systems. So why don't they behave in a way conducive to your well-being? The fact is, hospitals are in competition against each other (like businesses or institutions in other fields) and don't necessarily *want* to work together. This results in redundancy and waste, and can be detrimental to your health.

Institutions are also in competition in terms of research. Not only might they fail to discuss your ailment with each other, they may resist sharing research findings. There may be many researchers working on finding a cure for the same disease, but one hospital will decline to share its findings with another institution because they're both racing to discover it first. This kind of opposition can also be detrimental to patient health.

In general, free-market competition spurs innovation and keeps prices down. In the particular case of health care, however, it also creates redundancies that drive prices up. This is due to a lack of transparency about prices, making it impossible for patients to compare the costs of doctors, treatments, and hospital stays. To remedy this problem, President Donald Trump recently signed an executive order calling for price transparency so that consumers can see how much hospitals actually charge insurers. Transparency will force health care providers to stay competitive and will therefore help rein in costs. Of course, we also want competition to keep spurring the scientific community to continue researching and developing new medical technologies. If we can lower our costs by reducing redundancy and price gouging with improved transparency, we will offset the expected price increases from our future innovations.

Third-Party Profiteers

A huge part of our spending is on conditions that could be avoided with changes in our diet, lifestyle, and environmental factors. Those environmental factors include food choices—the vending machines in our office buildings, the kinds of restaurants and markets in our neighborhoods. People like to blame Big Food and Big Soda for tempting us. Then Big Pharma waits in the wings to give us a pill for the ailments we develop because of poor diets. Then people grumble about the rising costs of such treatments.

If a doctor does prescribe you a medication (which is very likely, whether you need it or not), you are the last stop on a long money train: pharmaceutical companies, insurance companies, pharmacy benefit managers, and pharmacies, all of them wanting a share of the profit.

The United Nations estimates that, by 2030, the estimated global economic toll of noncommunicable diseases—including cancer, cardiovascular disease, mental illness, and obesity-related illness—could reach $47 trillion. In the United States alone, four out of every five deaths are attributed to a noncommunicable disease.[2]

Naturally, Big Pharma wants to profit from those dollars. Because Big Pharma sees more money in long-term treatment, they develop and tout medications for conditions that could be prevented by changes in diet and lifestyle; they know most people will prefer to take a pill. They are betting against the American people, and they do so because they can count on us not to do the right thing for ourselves. If our goal is to be healthy and spend less on medical bills, and many of our illnesses are due to bad choices, why don't we tackle it at the source?

There is no conspiracy of physicians working for pharmaceutical corporations to keep you sick to result in big profits. The sad truth is, our need for instant gratification, for easy fixes, makes us more likely to take a medication than to change our behaviors.

Be Careful What You Ask For

Our amazing technological innovations in medicine can cost tens of millions of dollars to bring to market. It makes sense that state-of-the-art treatments would be expensive. Now, does that mean only the elite should have access to them? Of course not. But certainly the innovators and the investors who funded them should see a financial gain. We still have a capitalist system—at least for now. If we take away the financial incentive for innovation, we'll lose the venture capitalists who invest to help create new pharmaceuticals, artificial intelligence, and much more.

The United States has consistently taken the lead in developing vaccines, treatments, and cures for diseases such as cholera, chicken pox, polio, hepatitis, and AIDS. Today, people are living with HIV and hepatitis because of advanced medications. Just a few decades from the HIV and AIDS crisis, an HIV diagnosis is no longer a death sentence. In fact, some doctors would say they'd rather be diagnosed with HIV than type 2 diabetes—that's how manageable it is. We also have CAR T-cell therapy, a novel cancer treatment for childhood leukemia that is curing children. We identify problems and develop medicines to manage, and sometimes even cure, illnesses. In so many ways, the American health care story is a great success.

The point is we're not spending all this money for nothing in return. Despite its unnecessary complexity, the American medical system is worthy of envy in many categories, especially in cancer care. We have the shortest wait times and easiest access to new technology in the world, which is not limited to affluent and insured families. Likewise, if someone shows up to the emergency department having a heart attack, it doesn't matter if they have insurance or what their immigration status is; they'll still be treated immediately.

That's not the case everywhere outside of the United States. In one county in Britain, if you need a knee or hip replacement surgery but you're overweight or a smoker, you won't get the recommended surgery until you lose weight or quit. In other words, non-urgent care is to be rationed—saved primarily for those who demonstrate healthy behaviors. Some officials have warned that other parts of the NHS could start implementing these rules. To be honest, I don't completely disagree with that approach—it encourages healthier living. However, the rationing is not being done for altruistic reasons alone (i.e., to improve the health of citizens); it is driven by lack of funding and resources.[3] In the United States we will not ration your care. In fact, we will provide care no matter what shape patients are in, potentially to our own detriment.

Americans don't want to be told that we need to stop smoking or eat less red meat; we want the magic fix and we want it now. To a certain extent, we're getting exactly what we asked for—magic potions from doctors. Yes, our care costs more, but we want the potions. Then we complain about the ramifications and subsequent cost increases associated with our own demands.

Allowing Our Health Problems to Escalate

According to a 2017 study by the Kaiser Family Foundation, the United States has the highest rate of preventable deaths from heart attack, stroke, diabetes, cancer, overdoses, and suicides. So many things in our lives seem out of our hands—nuclear bomb threats, terrorist attacks, school shootings, horrible genetic diseases, car accidents. And yet we're not acting on the controllable factors in our lives. It's beyond shocking.

I am proud to be an American. I might not be proud of every detail of our history, but I love our founding principles. I'm grateful that I was not born in an oppressed nation and that I was given every opportunity not only as a female but also as a single teenage mother. And yes, I am proud that I took advantage of my opportunity to be successful. At the same time, I'm saddened when my fellow Americans take advantage of their freedom for the worse.

We're living free, and we're living longer, but we're hurting.

Where Do We Go from Here?

As people live longer, we are also living longer with chronic illnesses. Even though we shell out more money on health care than any other country in the world, the CDC says that 75 percent of those dollars go toward chronic conditions. Almost half of American adults have a chronic condition. What is even more troubling is that chronic conditions are on the rise among *all* age groups, not just adults. One in five adults has arthritis—the most common cause of disability in America—which is largely linked to lifestyle and weight. Children have higher obesity rates than ever before.[4] Consequently we're seeing a huge rise in teenagers with type 2 diabetes. Before the obesity epidemic in our country, type 2 diabetes was practically unheard of in people under 30; that's why it was formerly called adult-onset diabetes. Reports from the CDC predict that one in three children born in the year 2000 in the United States will develop type 2 diabetes in their lifetimes unless there are significant changes in diet and physical-activity levels.

We are living in an "obesogenic" environment of processed and fast food, and it is taking its toll on children. Schools are not placing enough importance on physical education and activity. Parents can easily sign a waiver for their child to opt out of any physical activity during school for various reasons. When children are at home, parents are too afraid to let them play outside or climb a tree or walk or ride bikes on their own. Children (like their parents) are glued to their devices. The massive influx of screen technology has also created newly recognized forms of depression and anxiety and pushed children and adults alike further from direct human interaction and physical activity.

We are afraid to call out problems of obesity and sedentariness because we are afraid of being considered prejudiced or mean. We can't talk about obesity for fear of being accused of "fat shaming." When the American Academy of Pediatrics put out a statement on the increasing obesity rates among children, it recommended approaching the topic using neutral words like "weight" and "body-mass index" rather than "obese," "fat," or "weight problem."

This is not to say that we should use weight stigmatization or shaming to motivate people to lose weight. Rather than motivate positive change, the stigma associated with being overweight can actually contribute to damaging behaviors such as binge eating, social isolation, avoidance of medical services, decreased physical activity, and increased long-term weight gain. So, yes, stigma is something to be concerned about. However, in our desire to avoid stigma, have we traveled too far in the other direction, protecting emotions instead of determining solutions to the problem? Of course we don't want to emotionally damage anyone; we just want them to be healthier! All of these factors combined have kept us from stating the truth: we are spiraling downward because of our own actions.

If we don't change our trajectory, we are going to continue suffering from our most common (and in many cases preventable) ailments: heart attacks, strokes, and cancer. If we're not careful, as is happening with type 2 diabetes and certain mental-health disorders, our children will start suffering from even more adult illnesses.

Then their children—our grandchildren—will suffer further. Considering where we are now, imagine how bankrupt the system will be for our grandchildren. They may not have the resources to break *our* bad habits.

We Are the Problem

Undoubtedly, the American health care system has its issues and inefficiencies, but it is also one of the most innovative and accessible systems in the world. We shouldn't discourage investors from taking interest in those innovations, and we can't avoid the fact that making medical advances is expensive. Free-market competition alone won't help us out of this mess, but it's going to play a critical role. A national government takeover would halt technological progress in the medical sector. Shouldn't we instead take action as individuals to decrease the costs we *can* control?

According to the Partnership to Fight Chronic Disease (PFCD), "more than 190 million Americans, or about 59 percent of the population, are affected by one or more chronic diseases." In 2016 the PFCD warned that, by 2030, the overall cost of chronic diseases in America alone was projected to reach $42 trillion.[5] Rather than trusting the government to find a solution to our mess, is there an alternative way to decrease this financial, emotional, and physical burden? *We* as individuals and as a society have the power to decrease prices and the prevalence of illnesses—not by making a pill less expensive, or by cutting the cost of physician visits, but by changing our own behaviors to decrease the demand. If we cut overall expenses by taking steps to avoid diseases that are in fact avoidable, we will continue to be a world leader in medical innovations, and ultimately our health care system will be more accessible, more affordable, and more efficient.

The only way we can change the system is if Americans change their mind-set and admit that we are all part of the problem.

Chapter 3

AMERICA, YOU'RE BREAKING OUR HEART

Most of us take our heart for granted—beating away, every minute pumping 1.5 gallons of blood through the body. Think of the work that this powerful muscle puts in every single minute. Yet we pay no attention to it until the emergency alarms go off. Not paying attention has a high cost: cardiovascular disease is the number one killer in the United States and worldwide.

Often referred to as heart disease, cardiovascular disease is an umbrella term for a group of problems that occur when the heart and/or blood vessels aren't working the way they should. It includes several conditions, with the most common in the United States being coronary artery disease, which affects the small arteries that supply blood to the heart muscle. Decreased blood flow in the coronary arteries can ultimately lead to a heart attack. Heart disease also puts you at risk of stroke, caused by decreased blood flow in the vessels to the brain.

Despite the known risk factors for heart disease, many Americans remain complacent. Some are not even familiar with the everyday culprits increasing their risk of disease. As if our own complacency were not bad enough, every year that we live increases the risk for heart disease. As I've said, we keep consuming

foods and beverages that are bad for our health, as the corporations who produce them profit off our poor choices.

This chapter offers a refresher on recognizing risk factors and
understanding how behaviors affect health. It also provides a few
tips on what you can do to take charge of your heart health. It
covers the various obstacles Americans face in stewarding their
health—from the corporate producers of food and drink to over-
reliance on a generous welfare state.

The Seat Belt for Your Heart

In 1945 the unexpected death of President Franklin Delano Roosevelt from a stroke prompted new awareness of the dangers of
cardiovascular disease. Roosevelt suffered from hypertension (high
blood pressure) and heart disease, but the public was not told how
serious his condition was. At the time little treatment was available
other than bed rest. In 1948, three years after FDR's death, Congress passed the National Heart Act, which created a new National
Heart Institute focusing on research into cardiovascular disease.

The National Heart Act resulted in the Framingham Heart
Study, which revolutionized our approach toward diseases like
high blood pressure and cardiovascular disease. Before this study,
physicians viewed these illnesses as an inevitable consequence
of aging. But after the study was released, it became obvious that
these diseases were largely a result of lifestyle factors that could be
altered to avoid such a diagnosis.[1]

The increase in life expectancy in the United States paradoxi-
cally led to an increase in the prevalence of heart disease. Heart
disease was less common not because people were healthier but
because people died at younger ages from something else. Living
longer does not necessarily result in heart disease, but the com-

bination of a longer life and certain lifestyle choices does significantly increase our risk of developing cardiovascular disease.
Heart disease has long been considered a man's disease, but the
same number of men and women die of it in the United States
every year.

Effective Scare Tactics

Imagine if we took precautions to maintain the health of our hearts
as we do for other things. For example, to avoid unsightly signs
of aging, I diligently apply sunscreen, use Retin-A topical facial
cream, and, between you and me, get occasional Botox injections.
I'm careful with the food I eat (though I could eat more vegetables),
knowing that I have a difficult time making it to the gym as
frequently as I should with my work and family schedule. I also
average about two glasses of wine per week, which approaches the
limit of the recommended amount. Despite my less-than-stringent
health regimen, I am one of the healthy ones because I maintain a
reasonably balanced diet and some level of physical activity.

The bottom line is that we don't necessarily have to make a drastic
change to move toward a healthier self. Rather, small, manageable
changes may be all anyone needs. Why haven't we as a nation fig-
ured this out? Do we really need the government to take charge of
our lives the way a parent watches over a child?

Imagine buying a car without seat belts—or getting into a car
and not buckling up for safety. We do it without thinking. But this
wasn't always the case. It wasn't until the 1960s that seat belts were
required in all US autos and not until the 1980s that states began passing laws requiring their use. After a mostly unsuccessful
"buckle up" ad campaign, in the 1980s the National Ad Council
and the Department of Transportation's National Highway Traffic

Safety Administration ran an ad campaign that was finally effective in getting Americans to buckle up. Mandated use of seat belts by drivers and front-seat passengers has reduced the risk of death by 45 percent and cut the risk of serious injury by 50 percent.[2] It is sad to say, but it took the threat of getting ticketed and having to pay a fine to compel people to make the right decisions for their own safety on the road.

So what does this tell us about persuading Americans to start protecting their cardiovascular health? According to the CDC, at least one million American deaths each year could be prevented.[3] More than half of those deaths involve people under the age of sixty-five. The death rate from car accidents went down after the decades-long effort to encourage commonsense use of seat belts, but far too many people are still dying from a disease that other commonsense precautions could prevent. This isn't just true of our elderly population. This affects everyone.

The American Heart Association and Centers for Disease Control reports on cardiovascular disease found that about 80 percent of deaths from heart disease can be attributed to an individual's lifestyle.[4] Can you imagine if we determined a way to modify lifestyle factors to reduce those affected by cardiovascular disease to merely 20 percent of our current burden? Why are we so slow to adopt the proper measures? Do we in fact need the government to step in as they did with seat belt laws? Is that really what we've come to, that we require our government—like the county health council in Britain that decided obese people and smokers would be denied surgeries—to force us to take care of ourselves? I hope not.

For many people, dying in a plane crash strikes fear into their hearts, yet there's only one fatal accident for every 16 million commercial airline flights. Meanwhile, more than one person in the United States dies every minute of every day from a heart disease–

related event.[5] Let that number sink in for a minute. Why isn't there an equivalent fear of heart disease? My theory is that we are more likely to be afraid of things outside our control than of things within our control.

YOUR CHOICES ADD UP

Although children don't usually have symptoms of heart disease, we need to introduce them to healthy habits while they're still young. Young adults (ages 24 to 29) with common risk factors such as smoking, obesity, and high cholesterol have a 25 percent higher risk of experiencing significant narrowing of coronary arteries than young adults without those risk factors. Narrower arteries decrease blood flow and thus the oxygen the heart requires to pump effectively.

Enemy Number One: Your Diet

Poor diets are associated with nearly one in five American deaths. A poor diet is one that is high in trans fats and sugary drinks and low in whole grains, vegetables, fruits, nuts, and fish oil.[6] Want to know what *really* happens when you eat some of America's favorite unhealthy foods and don't exercise? Let's take a brief look inside your blood to understand.

When we regularly consume processed foods (potato chips, breakfast cereals, most white bread) and sugary drinks (soda and fruit juice) and lead a sedentary lifestyle, along with other bad habits, we get a buildup of plaque in our blood vessels. The blood vessels are an intricate highway system throughout the body, and plaque from poor eating habits acts as debris blocking the road. Plaque buildup results in a massive traffic slowdown that would make the New Jersey Turnpike commute look easy. This restriction of flow is what causes cardiovascular disease, resulting in heart disease, heart attacks, peripheral vascular disease, kidney failure, dementia, and strokes, to name a few ailments.

Think about one of America's biggest weaknesses: fried food. Most such foods are made with processed vegetable oils like canola oil. Packaged cookies, cakes, and other processed sweets are loaded with sugar. Both of these contribute to plaque buildup in our arteries.

What about the quintessential American holiday, the Fourth of July? It's the day we all get together to celebrate and enjoy a healthy spread of salads, grilled fish, fruit, and water . . . right? Not exactly. We're a lot more likely to gorge on hot dogs and processed meats, full of unhealthy fats, on processed white-bread buns. Then we fill up our plates with potato chips and potato or pasta salad—all containing refined white starch. All of these foods serve as a rocket boost to blood sugar and cholesterol. Don't forget the beer, soda, or sweetened iced tea. Although beer has a few minor health benefits, let's be honest: the main effects are a belly and a few extra pounds. How about berry desserts with sugary crusts and processed whipped topping? More carbs, more sugar, more garbage.

If we spend most days eating health-consciously, then there's nothing wrong with enjoying a holiday splurge. Believe me—I do! The problem is that so many people eat like this regularly—and more often than they want to admit.

One hot dog is not going to cause high blood pressure or high cholesterol. Even if you want to splurge once a week, that's better than having it every day. The goal is to find a balance. We don't all need to become vegans or juicer fanatics or adopt the latest fad diet. I'm only asking you to limit consumption of unhealthy foods and eat healthier counterparts more often.

The Big Food and Drink Industry Takeover

Regular consumption of highly processed foods like hot dogs, potato chips, sugary cereals, processed meats, packaged cookies, and sugary drinks has been proven repeatedly to be directly linked to obesity and obesity-related diseases like diabetes and cardiovascular disease. What about some popular foods that are advertised as healthy but in fact also contribute to our poor health, such as microwave popcorn, fruit juice, low-fat flavored yogurt, dried fruit, smoothies, and even many gluten-free products?

Let me explain: food companies make food tastier by adding salt and sugar; they make it last longer with artificial preservatives. Microwave popcorn is low in calories but can be loaded with sodium and preservatives. People thought low-fat yogurt was supposed to be better for you than full-fat yogurt, but to make the low-fat yogurt taste good, the yogurt brands added more sugar to it. People knew soda was bad for you so they grabbed a bottle of "all-natural" juice instead, not realizing it has the same amount of sugar as soda, or sometimes even more. (For that reason, pediatricians have stopped recommending juice for children.) Similarly, many people eat dried fruit because it's fruit. Isn't that supposed to be healthy? Unfortunately, dried fruit, although high in fiber, is also quite high in sugar and calories. A little is okay, but it's not necessarily a healthy snack. Big Food found ways to maintain profits by marketing these foods as healthy, while consumers started seeing their waistlines expand.

Americans' average body-mass index, or BMI (a measure of

body fat in adults based on height and weight), has increased over the years.[7] The rising rate of obesity, in turn, has contributed to a rise in cardiovascular disease. In fact, approximately 121 million American adults live with some form of cardiovascular disease.

Cardiovascular disease doesn't just affect the clinically obese (those with a BMI of 30 or more) but also the larger population of people who are marginally overweight (those with a BMI between 25 and 29.9)—those who don't necessarily consider their weight to be a health risk. "Marginally overweight" is the blissful place of ignorance where so many Americans live. Although the health risks are more severe for those considered obese, even marginally overweight people are at risk for developing all the maladies we are discussing, all of which not only cost our nation billions of dollars annually but also result in a poor quality of life and premature death.

Unfortunately, for many people it is easier to take a magic pill to thwart the effects of chronic disease than to make lifestyle modifications. Too many people cannot—or will not, rather—give up their daily high-sugar mochas. The good news is this: *even a small amount of weight loss, and any increase in physical activity, immediately lowers the risk of developing disease.*

I believe that most people *want* to change but are stuck in habits that go back all the way to childhood, especially when it comes to diet. Old habits may die hard, but change is worth it for your health and well-being.

Enemy Number Two: Tobacco

A 2012 government study showed that almost half of all Americans have at least one of the three key risk factors for heart disease: high blood pressure, high cholesterol, and smoking.[8] Although a family history may contribute to the first two, smoking is exclusively by choice.

Smoking tobacco not only damages the heart and blood vessels, but it also increases the risk of many resulting conditions, like heart attack, aneurysms, and strokes. The nicotine alone in cigarettes raises blood pressure by narrowing the vessels (so, yes, vaping nicotine products does this too). Moreover, the carbon monoxide in some cigarettes reduces the amount of oxygen that blood can carry. Even simple exposure to other people's secondhand smoke increases the risk for heart and lung disease because of the toxicities in the smoke.

Much like a poor diet, there is nothing to gain from smoking, and everything to lose from it.

Despite all of the known harms, the marketing efforts of Big Tobacco lured us into thinking that smoking is fun, sexy, relaxing, and cool. Even today, after anti-smoking efforts have revealed the truth about smoking, cigarettes still conjure images of stylish Parisian women smoking at a cafe or James Dean smoking while sitting on a motorcycle.

Despite the cultural associations, there is nothing attractive about tobacco-induced heart disease. Since the 1960s, the US government, as well as state and local governments, has made concerted efforts to educate and warn the public about the dangers of smoking, especially by pregnant women and minors. High taxes on cigarettes, restrictions on tobacco ads, warning labels on tobacco products, and graphic public service announcements showing the ravages of smoking-related disease on the body have all helped bring down the numbers of Americans who smoke. Smoking is banned on public transportation, in or near schools, in many privately owned buildings and an array of business establishments. There has been much progress. Yet 14 out of every 100 adults in the United States still smoke cigarettes.[9]

My husband is an endovascular neurosurgeon. He performs

lifesaving surgeries on people every day for conditions such as brain tumors, stroke, and brain aneurysms. Brain aneurysms—a ruptured blood vessel in the brain, often caused by smoking and high blood pressure—carry a 45 percent mortality rate. Of those who survive a rupture, 65 percent suffer from a permanent neurological deficit. All too often, his patients smoke tobacco. Without time for consideration, he intervenes to save their lives when he gets the urgent phone call. If they survive and become stable, he discusses with them a plan to improve their health that includes diet, exercise, and smoking cessation.

At times, during a follow-up appointment several months later, patients will return and report that they have not made changes to their lifestyle. They have narrowly escaped death, and yet they refuse to forgo the habits that put them in that situation in the first place. Should we refer to patients like this as "victims" of disease? Their ailments are a direct result of their intentional bad habits, which they maintain even after a near-death emergency. As a physician, I view all my patients as victims of disease, regardless of cause. Everyone deserves treatment and empathy as they are suffering. But the issue of preventable illness does cause one to wonder: Who should be responsible for the long-term financial consequences of the chronic disease directly caused by intentional choice? As a society we collectively pay for these illnesses; so do we all become victims?

The cost associated with smoking-related illness by the 14 percent of Americans who smoke cigarettes, in addition to those affected by their secondhand smoke, is as much as $170 billion annually.[10] No wonder our health care costs are skyrocketing and individuals with high-cost medical bills are forced into bankruptcy. Should the responsible, nonsmoking 86 percent of the adult population contribute to this expense when there is ample warning not to use cigarettes?

Some people even have the audacity to say, "I'm not going to quit smoking. I enjoy it too much." And in response, physicians will ponder, "Why should I perform this procedure on you? Why should the insurance company be charged? Why should other people pay for the harm you inflict on your own body?"

Nobody ever has a good answer. Prior to the Affordable Care Act, insurance premiums were higher for smokers, which seems rational given that the likelihood of disease in a smoker is far greater than in a nonsmoker. Yet now we continue like a cog in the wheel going around without holding people accountable for choices that result in (expensive) diseases.

Enemy Number Three: Refusing Medication

In the United States, there are about 3.8 billion prescriptions written every year.[11] As you might imagine, doctors are prescribing a lot of medication for our hearts. Yet, according to various studies, roughly 50 percent of those prescriptions are taken incorrectly or not taken at all. Moreover, 20 to 30 percent are never even filled at the pharmacy.[12] Compared to the patients who follow their physician's advice and take their medications appropriately, the patients who don't take their medications as intended have significant risks of hospitalization, readmission to the hospital, and premature death.

I find it hard to understand why patients with serious cardiac conditions don't take their medication. Here's how the conversation generally goes: The doctor tells the patient, you have a health problem. I'm prescribing a medication that, in addition to lifestyle changes, is going to help fix the problem. If you don't take it, there's a chance you will die. The patient leaves the hospital and, despite having this knowledge, chooses not to take the medicine. It's a confusing phenomenon.

The former surgeon general C. Everett Koop once said, "Drugs don't work on people who don't take them." As physicians, we can only prescribe so much, and pharmaceutical companies can only develop so much. At a certain point, patients must take control of their own fate and make choices to save their lives. Why do people not take medications as prescribed? Is the medication too expensive? Did the patient develop side effects? Or did they just not want to take it? It's a combination of all three. The cost of medicine is a major reason for noncompliance, but even when patients are given the drugs for free, compliance improves only slightly. Patients don't take their medications for a multitude of reasons, many of which we may never understand. Our reasons for our decisions are as complex as we are. When it comes to chronic disease, people often just don't feel sick—what they don't seem to understand is that they must take their medication to *avoid* the consequences of the disease and premature death.

A lack of medication adherence causes nearly 125,000 deaths each year. Nonadherence also causes 10 percent of all hospitalizations, costing our already strained health care system anywhere between $100 to $289 billion annually.[13]

My husband treated a middle-aged man recently who led an unhealthy lifestyle: he smoked two packs of cigarettes a day, was overweight, and self-admittedly did not exercise. As a result, he developed a form of cardiovascular disease in the large vessels carrying blood to his brain. His condition required a stent (a small tube placed in an artery after it has closed from plaque buildup to keep the blood vessel open and improve blood flow to the vital organ). Anytime someone has a foreign object, like a stent, implanted in the body, the body wants to reject it and protect itself from it, even if it is there to help. To compensate for that phenomenon, when someone undergoes this lifesaving intervention, often they must be on certain medications afterward to prevent the rejection and failure of the device.

This gentleman was prescribed two medications to do just that, both of which prevent blood from clotting and attacking the stent. However, for no reported reason, the man decided he didn't want to take his medication. There was no obvious barrier to cost. He did not report any side effects. He would take the medication occasionally, but he didn't make it part of his daily routine.

What happened? The stent shut down and he suffered a major stroke. He had been told this could happen if he did not take the medications, yet he refused to do so. My husband left our anniversary dinner to go and save the man's life again—but the damage to the brain had been done. Not only had the stent failed, but he had waited too long to go to the hospital, which resulted in brain damage from the lack of oxygen. Now being cared for by his family, he can no longer work. His choice not to take his medication drastically decreased his own quality of life and that of his family. His choice also abruptly put an end to the contributions he was making or might have made, through work or otherwise, to society. Our individual choices have long-term societal consequences.

My Insurance Will Cover This

Each day in the hospital I witness a troubling pattern: Highly specialized physicians are called on to perform lifesaving procedures. Their heroic efforts often lead to happy outcomes. Yet these fortunate patients often find out later that their insurance company has denied payment for the intervention that was performed.

Deny, deny, deny—that's the modus operandi of insurance companies. They come up with whatever possible reason to deny coverage. They rationalize the rejection with something as ridiculous as, "We will cover the CT scan, but not the doctor's fee for the radiologist who interprets the images." Or they say, "There is not enough evidence-based medicine to prove this treatment works." Even if an intervention resulted in a successful outcome and the patient is thriving, the insurance company may still ultimately refuse to pay for it. Imagine that—the surgery did, in fact, save the patient's life, but the claim is denied because there's not enough research to prove it works. *Sigh*. The financial burden subsequently placed on the patient (not to mention the lack of reimbursement to the physician and medical personnel) can be overwhelming, even resulting in bankruptcy.

Although nobody should be forced to declare bankruptcy because of a nonelective medical procedure, people go too far in the other direction: they don't want to pay *anything* for their care. There are countless services we willingly pay for—a haircut, an oil change on our car, the latest smartphone. But when a doctor performs a medically necessary procedure, some people believe it is a "right" to receive that service without shouldering some of the cost, whether or not they can afford it.

Of course, not every claim gets denied. Insurance companies *do* pay out large sums for the treatment of various diseases, including preventable ones. Insurance companies, like hospitals and doctors, also have bottom lines. So premiums go up, or coverage gets restricted in other ways. We seem to be stuck: we assume our insurance will cover everything and are shocked when it doesn't. Yet we're unwilling to change our behaviors to stay healthy and thereby avoid some of the ballooning costs of medical care and health insurance. As long as insurance companies continue to foot the bill for diseases that are potentially preventable, there is little financial incentive for patients to quit the lifestyle pattern that put them in medical danger in the first place.

Where's the sense in all of this? Unfortunately, our heated political debates haven't brought us any closer to workable solutions. But solutions do exist.

Solutions

We must get to the root of the problem and start preventing disease before irreversible damage occurs. The self-inflicted damage is sentencing us to a lifetime of expensive medications and doctors' visits. My advice is simple: Don't smoke, maintain a healthy weight through conscious nutrition (including at least five servings of fruits and vegetables daily), and get at least 150 minutes of any level of exercise each week. If you do these three things and still can't get to where you need to be in terms of blood pressure, cholesterol, and weight, take the medication prescribed by your doctor. It isn't a sign of moral failure to need medication. We are only able to control so much; our genetic makeup may require more than diet and lifestyle changes.

Stop making excuses about why you can't. Your spouse, children, friends, co-workers, and everyone else around you depend on you. Not to mention the health care costs you're driving up for everybody. Be a good neighbor to us all—get an annual medical checkup, put down the cigarette, walk away from the fried foods, and take a walk around the block.

Making decisions like these will change your life for the better. Your chances of developing heart disease and cancer will plummet. And yes, I did say cancer. Contrary to public opinion, many cancers also fall well within the realm of preventable disease and can be avoided with the same lifestyle changes prescribed for heart disease.

Chapter 4

THE BIG C: CANCER

Heart disease kills more Americans than any other disease, but cancer is right behind it. According to the National Cancer Institute, men and women have approximately a 39 percent chance of being diagnosed with cancer in their lifetimes.[1] In some areas of the country, cancer is gaining ground: in 2014, twenty-two states had more cancer deaths than heart disease deaths. That was a substantial and troubling increase from 2002, when only two states had more cancer deaths than heart disease deaths.[2]

Like heart disease, many cancers are preventable. Let me say that again because this rarely sinks in for people: *Nearly half of all cancer diagnoses may be preventable.*

We often react to cancer as an overwhelming diagnosis, but it doesn't have to be. Not only can we improve our odds of never getting the disease, but we can also diminish its impact if we do get a diagnosis of the Big C.

Understanding Cancer

Similar to cardiovascular disease, the word "cancer" is an extremely broad term for a large group of diseases that can affect any part of the body. One defining feature of cancer is a rapid growth and spread of abnormal cells. When cells grow outside of their usual boundaries, like weeds in a garden, they can invade neighboring parts of the body and spread to other organs.

As a category of disease, cancer causes one in four deaths. The American Cancer Society estimated that, in the United States in 2019, there would be 1,660 deaths from cancer every day, and just over 600,000 deaths from cancer over the course of the year.[3]

One-third of all Americans are going to develop cancer at some point in their lifetime.[4] The most common type of cancer is non-melanoma skin cancer, such as squamous- and basal-cell cancers. Next on the list are breast, lung, prostate, colon, stomach, and liver cancers.

Cancer can form anywhere in the body, from head to toe, because our bodies are made of trillions of cells. As our cells age and die normally, our body produces new cells to replace them with safety checks along the way to make sure everything forms appropriately. When there is a breakdown in this process, either the damaged cells continue to proliferate or new abnormal cells grow. This is when cancer develops. The disruption in the safety check process can be caused by a multitude of factors either acting alone or in conjunction with other variables.

Our own genetic makeup (DNA) may predispose us to form some cancers. Public awareness of genetic susceptibility has increased drastically thanks to prominent news stories, such as those about Angelina Jolie's BRCA mutation and about home genetic testing by companies like 23andMe. Although those stories make the headlines, only 5 to 10 percent of all cancers are caused by inherited genetic mutations. The rest happen because of the damage we expose our bodies to throughout our lifetime. Yes, often we do it to ourselves.

Normal aging is a fundamental factor. The incidence of cancer rises dramatically with age, likely due to a lifetime buildup of physical, chemical, and biological carcinogenic exposure. The overall risk accumulates, and as we age, our bodies lose the ability to repair themselves.

WHAT ARE CARCINOGENS?

A carcinogen is a cancer-causing substance. Physical carcinogens are things such as ultraviolet (UV) rays (the reason we wear hats and sunscreen) and ionizing radiation (think hazard signs outside of the x-ray room). Some chemical carcinogens include asbestos, toxic chemicals associated with tobacco intake, and arsenic.

The great news is that the number of people living beyond their cancer diagnosis is getting higher every day. As of early 2019, that number reached 16.9 million people, and it's expected to rise to almost 121.7 million by 2029.[5] These days, when I tell my patients they have cancer, I can immediately follow that by telling them the chances are, within a year from the day of diagnosis, they will have put treatment behind them and be able to get on with their lives. There is a lot of good news to celebrate in the fight against cancer. Research by the American Cancer Society shows that the death rate from cancer in the United States actually decreased by 27 percent from 1991 to 2016.[6] Much of the drop is due to reduced rates of smoking, as well as earlier detection through screenings and improvements in cancer treatments.

People would have thought you were insane if you said this fifty years ago, but here it is: we are now able to treat cancer as a chronic disease, similar to diabetes and heart disease. If you get cancer, yes, you'll likely have lifelong medical care—but it doesn't necessarily mean your life will be cut short. In fact, you may die from heart disease or another illness long before your cancer becomes life-threatening.

However, one new problem we face with all of these miraculous treatment methods is that cancer care is expensive, and it's even more expensive when it's diagnosed at a later stage.

The Costs of Illness and Innovation

Cancer's effects extend far beyond the individual with cancer and his or her family. It also affects us as a society. According to the National Cancer Institute, in 2010 the United States spent $157 billion in cancer care. That figure is projected to surpass $174 billion in 2020.[7] What this number does not include is the subsequent lost revenue from cancer patients not being able to work, either permanently or temporarily, because of their disease. The total annual economic cost of cancer through health care expenditure plus loss of productivity is approximately $1.2 trillion per year.[8]

An amazing new leukemia treatment called CAR T-cell therapy is curing children of the deadly disease. This is a huge breakthrough, but it's a very expensive medication, costing about $100,000 per dose. Considering that hardly any patients are able to pay for it, what good is it? If insurance companies cover this treatment, then premiums will have to go up. If the government pays for it, taxpayers are footing the bill. So, who should pay for it? These are difficult questions. This is just one example of the ethical and practical dilemmas of determining how to deal with the cost of advancing care.

It is expensive to have nearly any disease, but cancer treatments can have huge costs. Many of the treatments are covered by insurance plans, but patients often have substantial out-of-pocket costs. Add to that financial strain the potential loss of income from days away from work. There is another cost of illness, one borne by everyone: reduced or loss of income for people with serious illness in turn means fewer dollars being paid to the government in taxes.

Costs also go up when people delay getting help. We tend to wait for that emergency alarm to sound before we do something to save ourselves, as with heart disease. I see it all the time with breast cancer patients.

The United States has the most robust breast cancer screening programs in the world. Yet in any given year, up to 50 percent of American women do not get the mammograms recommended based on their age or risk factors. The reasons vary, ranging from lack of time, to discomfort of the mammogram, to being afraid of the results. My grandmother died from advanced breast cancer because she was too modest to go to her male doctor for any issue related to her breast. She also skipped her screening mammograms for the same reason, so she gave up any chance of diagnosing her cancer at an earlier stage. Today, we have much-improved tests for catching many cancers early, especially breast cancer—there's no excuse not to get tested. Women who don't get screening mammograms and clinical breast exams are increasing the risk of a delayed diagnosis of a treatable disease.

The chances of dying from certain cancers have drastically decreased with our latest therapies and screening modalities. The risk of death is not eliminated entirely, but treatment of a cancer at stage III versus stage I is not only more invasive and arduous for the patient, but it's also incredibly more expensive. Research has shown that "the average costs allowed per patient in the 24 months after the index diagnosis were $71,909, $97,066, $159,442, and $182,655 for disease stage 0, I/II, III, and IV, respectively."[9] A late-stage diagnosis also means their survival is reduced, so the treatments are more costly for fewer years gained.

What could have been a less dangerous surgery at an early stage turns into a complex operation at a later stage, plus radiation, chemotherapy, and other potential treatments. When patients become proactive with their recommended cancer screenings, they are potentially saving themselves a lot of heartache and, frankly, money, while also avoiding contributing to rising health care costs for all.

Of course, there are cancers that are unpreventable, as well as many for which there is no good screening mechanism, making early detection difficult. Some cancers occur no matter what you do to avoid them, and you can't do anything about it. Shouldn't these be the cases that we focus our resources on, both to expand research and to help those suffering? Unfortunately, our ability to concentrate on the unavoidable diagnoses is diluted by the 30 to 60 percent of cancers that could possibly have been avoided.

To Pay or Not to Pay

In addition to prevention and early detection, every year we're developing more advanced cancer treatments. For example, we now target DNA with precision medicine. Traditional methods like chemotherapy poison the cancer, but chemo also damages perfectly healthy cells in the process, leaving many patients with lifelong complications. With precision medicine, we're going in and turning the repair genes (safety checks) back on so our own body can fight the cancer.

However, there is an alarming trend in cancers today. When it comes to delivering a cancer diagnosis, the elephant in the room is whether or not there were clear extrinsic risk factors for the disease. In February 2019 research by the American Cancer Society demonstrated that, among adults under fifty, the rates of cancer directly linked to obesity are increasing. Even more startling is that younger populations are at a greater risk of developing certain cancers. Millennials (born between 1981 and 1996) are now twice as likely to develop six types of cancer as were baby boomers (born between 1946 and 1964) at the same age. As a mother of three, I find this terrifying. I should also point out that this is the generation that is rallying for government-subsidized health care (along with free college tuition, college-loan debt forgiveness, and guaranteed basic income). Perhaps they know their generation's medical costs are going to be higher than at any time in the nation's history, so they are asking early on for handouts.

Let me present two scenarios, both of which concern patients I have diagnosed. The first is a thirty-two-year-old woman who went to her ob-gyn because of an enlarging abdomen and pain. After a physical exam, ultrasound, MRI, blood work, and abdominal surgery, she was diagnosed with an aggressive ovarian cancer. Genetic testing revealed that she was born with a DNA mutation inherited from her father.

The second scenario is a fifty-two-year-old woman who went to her doctor because she had blood in her urine. The first question the doctor asked her was whether she ever smoked cigarettes. Smokers are four to seven times more likely to develop bladder cancer than nonsmokers. When she answered that she had smoked a pack of cigarettes every day for the last thirty years, he ordered a CT scan (in addition to a urine test), which led to a diagnosis of bladder cancer.

In the American health system, both of these patients receive the best available treatments regardless of what factors contributed to their cancers. My role as a physician is to care for all my patients equally; all patients are human beings deserving of respect and the best that medicine has to offer, whether or not they might have prevented their disease. However, this nondiscriminatory practice, to which I am committed, may be enabling our problem: preventable diseases are burdening our system and forcing us toward rationed health care.

It's one thing to love thy neighbor. However, it may be something completely different to take responsibility for your neighbor's self-destruction.

The Price of Innovation

As our nation gets older, cancer is going to continue to become more prevalent. As a result, we will have more cancer survivors. Even when there is no cure, most cancers can be controlled. It's amazing that people will be alive to seek further treatment, but that's still a huge strain on the economy.

Cancer research leading to innovations in testing and treatment is largely financed by venture capitalists, coupled with funding by the National Institutes of Health (NIH). That's how America works: private entities partnering with government, as well as charitable organizations, to advance medicine. Private companies have invested hundreds of millions of dollars to develop a variety of innovative therapies.

Pharmaceutical companies spend an estimated $2.6 billion on developing new prescription drugs that gain marketing approval, according to a 2016 study by the Tufts Center for the Study of Drug Development. The Trump administration has moved to decrease the average time it takes to bring a drug through clinical trials. However, the success rate for new drugs has gone down by almost half:

just 12 percent prove safe and effective enough to make it to market, after billions of dollars are spent and drug companies risk going belly up.[10] The pharmaceutical companies and their investors are left with a deficit of dollars and time invested in failed products.

When a drug does pass through the innumerable hoops to prove it is safe and effective, the pharmaceutical companies must make up for the losses of their prior failed endeavors, so they charge an inflated price for the one therapy that makes it. They also want to maximize profit while the new drug is under patent; after the patent expires, a competitor can manufacture a generic version that will cost far less. Headlines will declare that a medicine is too expensive for anyone to afford, and this is often true. However, prices listed publicly are hardly what the actual medicine costs or what any insurance plan or person will ever pay for it.

As Americans, we know that competition and the profit motive often drive innovation, and we support the idea that companies should be compensated for their investment in developing a new drug. I will also go so far as to say they deserve a handsome profit for their creation. But how much is too much? Is there such a thing? My personal opinion is that originators and those who work hard should not be capped at their potential for profit. Yet do pharmaceutical CEOs need to be making tens of millions of dollars while middle-class Americans are paying high prices for the medications? To take just one example, it was reported that the CEO of biotech firm Regeneron had a compensation package of $47.5 million in 2016. If executive compensation in the industry continues to rise, will it stoke public resentment toward the free market? Will this resentment nudge us toward more government oversight? I believe it already has.

Some believe the government should place limits on the profits these companies make. Senator Bernie Sanders, who ran for the Democratic presidential nomination in 2016 and launched a second bid in 2019, suggests pharmaceutical and device companies be restricted to charging 120 percent above the cost of production. Does this factor in the losses accrued from failed products or is it just a magical number that feels right to him?

Modern-day socialists are claiming their plan is to contain costs on just about everything, but they are not developing a true solution to the fundamental problems. How can anyone suggest expanding access to a system that is already struggling to cover those currently in it? Health care cost containment without modifying overutilization sounds to me like a road to rationed medicine. The fact is, government price controls would be calamitous, focusing only on the supply side and doing nothing to get at the root of the problem, the excessive demand.

If we do shift into a single-payer health care system and let the government control pharmaceutical prices and profits, will we have less creation? Naturally we will. Our venture capital money won't go into miraculous drugs because there won't be as much revenue to be made in the pharmaceutical industry. The Trump administration, with the FDA, has taken steps toward reining in rising drug prices. Rather than regulating the free market by placing caps on prices, this administration is encouraging market competition and price transparency. By shortening the FDA approval process, limiting patent protections, and publicly criticizing egregious profiteering, the Trump administration is putting pressure on the pharmaceutical industry from a business-savvy point of view.

These simple steps may appear minor, but they are the changes that will keep prices down in the long term. More actions to encourage the free market will help us much more than asking the government to take over.

A national single-payer system would require increasing taxes and further borrowing to expand the current system. This concept ignores why health care in the United States is so expensive to begin with. Truly, additional taxing and regulation would only further obscure our greatest problem: preventable disease.

Knocking Down Risk Factors

What can we do to clean up this mess?

More than 1.7 million cancers were projected to be diagnosed in 2019 and at least 42 percent of them could have been prevented.[11] I don't mean they could have been prevented by living inside of a bubble or escaping to an island where you are not exposed to toxic substances, but rather by making simple changes to daily routines. Of the approximately 740,000 cases of preventable cancer diagnosed in 2019, over a third of them are from smoking tobacco. Given the known risks for smokers of developing cancer and/or heart disease and stroke, it is mind-boggling that nearly 34 million Americans, approximately 14 percent of all adults, are still smoking.[12] Controllable risk factors for cancer overlap to a surprising degree with those for cardiovascular disease: smoking cigarettes and a combination of poor eating habits, excess alcohol consumption, and physical inactivity.

Exercise

Adults need 150 minutes of moderate-intensity or 75 minutes of vigorous-intensity exercise each week. Kids should be getting 60 minutes per day. Their 20-minute school PE class or being on the playground just isn't enough.

Many of us live sedentary lifestyles, and it's not necessarily because we're lazy. That's just our culture. Most people sit at a desk for a solid eight hours a day. My day starts by getting my children ready for school, then driving an hour to work, working for nine hours without a formal break, driving an hour home, then making dinner, helping my kids with homework, and getting them ready for bed. By then, it's 8:00 p.m., and I'm completely exhausted, especially on days when I get up at 3:30 a.m. to make a TV appearance.

At what point in that day should I exercise? Honestly, I don't know. But I do know that I need to. I must make exercise a priority just like brushing my teeth and drinking water; it is all for the good of my health. Even if it's just taking twenty minutes out of work to do some jumping jacks and walk around the parking lot, I need to do it. So do you.

Moderate intensity doesn't have to mean sprinting on a treadmill or conquering the latest workout trend. Take a brisk walk on your lunch break. Play soccer outside with your kids or jump at the trampoline park with them rather than reading the latest news on your phone. Walk the half-mile to the store instead of driving. And, yes, it's time to stop using the drive-through every day . . . for everything.

Our children need more exercise, too. Over the past twenty years, an increased emphasis on standardized testing as a metric for student achievement and heightened awareness of bullying has led leaders in some states and school districts to cut recess time. Now children have more in-class instruction and decreased social interaction outside of the classroom.

Yet children need physical activity. As a parent, you must ask yourself a question: Are you willing to risk your child's physical well-being to protect them from hurt feelings? That's exactly what we're doing when we let them skip exercise to improve a test score or for fear of running up against playground bullies. Parents and teachers have to intervene when they see bullying take place, but depriving children of their only means of physical activity during the day is not the answer.

Diet

As we have seen, when our body-mass index gets too high, it often leads to cardiovascular disease. But it also affects our immune system, hormone levels, and cell growth. For example, once you start storing too much fat in your abdominal area, those fat cells can produce estrogen, in men and women. Estrogen is a risk factor for several cancers, including breast cancer. Among the other cancers that have been linked to a high BMI (over 25) are endometrial, liver, ovarian, and colon.

In general, a diet low in fruits and vegetables is another risk factor for cancer. Only one in ten Americans meets the recommended levels of fruit and vegetable consumption.

WHAT ARE PHYTOCHEMICALS?

Phytochemicals are naturally occurring plant chemicals that provide them with color, odor, and flavor. When we eat them, they can have positive effects on the chemical processes inside our bodies. In the simplest terms, these nutrients go into the bloodstream and suck up all the badness that wants to cause cancer. The vibrant colors of whole foods are nature's way of saying they are rich in vitamins, minerals, and phytochemicals. As noted by the CDC, "federal guidelines recommend that adults eat at least 1¹/₂ to 2 cups per day of fruit and 2 to 3 cups per day of vegetables."[13] To get my kids on the right track, I tell them to eat the colors of the rainbow.

Another risk factor for cancer is eating processed foods. Here's a simple test to figure out if a food is overly processed: if you look on the ingredients list and you can't pronounce the words, chances are that food contains artificial substances, including preservatives, and is therefore processed. (Some unpronounceable words on the label are, in fact, the scientific names of vitamins, but use this as a rule of thumb.) This category of food includes obvious items like candy that turns your tongue blue but also supposedly "healthy" canned soups.

Ultraprocessed foods have more calories, sodium, sugar, and fat than raw, unprocessed foods. People who live on ultraprocessed foods tend to be more overweight. Yet these foods are a growing part of Americans' diets. In 2016 a study found that 60 percent of calories in the average American's diet come from ultraprocessed foods.[14] More of the developing world is starting to eat this way, too. Leave it to America to lead the way in unhealthy eating.

Can we blame Big Food for our weight? They do line every aisle of the grocery store with inexpensive, ready-to-eat or easy-to-prepare processed foods. Or should we blame ourselves for not resisting them? Shouldn't we hold ourselves responsible for what we put in our mouths? We don't *have* to succumb to the brilliant marketing schemes of the food industry. Ultimately, it comes down to this: we need to take the time to evaluate what we're consuming, and realize that eating more nutritiously is in our control.

Food Addiction

It sounds crazy to say, but there is such a thing as food addiction.

Processed junk foods, full of sugars and starch, can have a powerful effect on the reward centers in our brains, where they trigger neurotransmitters like dopamine. Chocolate contains a variety of chemicals, some of which make us feel good by boosting our endorphins (the same chemicals released when you're exercising or having an orgasm). Chocolate may also boost serotonin levels that help us to feel relaxed. Those chemicals trigger an emotional response that you'll seek to re-create again and again, until you have a full-blown food addiction. At that point willpower is no match for the dopamine signal hijacking the biochemistry of the brain.

The fact that we may have food addictions isn't an excuse to indulge, but you don't have to feel guilty about satisfying your cravings. We all have them. Big Food tries to tempt all of us, and we end up behaving in ways we don't want to. Completely avoiding junk food might be impossible, because junk food, sadly, is a huge part of our society (work vending machines, waterparks, sporting events, movie theaters, and on and on). Ultimately though, it's we who decide whether we're going to give in to the cravings or not. We are in control of our actions.

Every day, a patient will tell me her cancer diagnosis convinced her to change her diet to improve her overall health. Here's my eternal question: *Why does it take a cancer diagnosis to prompt these changes?*

A balanced and diversified diet should be considered one of our top public-health priorities. If we focused on eating real food, we could not only improve our beach body, but we might just prevent cancer as well.

Alcohol

Alcohol is directly linked to mouth, esophageal, stomach, and liver cancers—in essence, everything alcohol touches on its way through your body is at risk of developing cancer. That's how toxic alcohol can be.

Many of us (yes, me too) enjoy drinking socially, but as a country, we are drinking far too much. Drinking beer is one of America's pastimes. Some of the most popular Super Bowl commercials every year are for beer companies. The ads are filled with beautiful people appearing to have a marvelous time thanks to the icy cold beer they're gripping. They don't ever appear to be drunk, and they never have beer bellies.

Enjoying everything in moderation is the key. If you can't control your consumption, you are risking your life because of it. There are guidelines for alcohol intake: women shouldn't exceed one drink a day, and men shouldn't exceed two. Anything more than that is considered excessive drinking, which substantially increases the risk of developing cancer. You can't skip having drinks for four days and then have five drinks on Friday—it doesn't work that way. If you insist on unwinding with alcohol after a day's work, then drink a single glass of red wine, which has natural antioxidants, and call it a night.

A Virus Can Cause Cancer?

More recently, certain viruses have also been confirmed to be just as likely to cause cancer as smoking tobacco. Human oncoviruses (cancer-causing viruses) account for an estimated 12 to 20 percent of cancers worldwide.[15] The most commonly known viruses are certain types of human papillomavirus (HPV), human immunodeficiency virus (HIV), hepatitis B and hepatitis C viruses, and Epstein-Barr virus (EBV).

HPV is the most common sexually transmitted virus in the

world and is present in up to 79 million Americans.[16] Women are often familiar with HPV because that's what their gynecologist looks for in a Pap smear. Nearly all cases of cervical cancer, and about 95 percent of anal cancers, are caused by an HPV infection. We are also finding that HPV plays a big role in mouth and throat cancers. The most troubling aspect of this virus is that it is an asymptomatic infection, so people are not aware they are infected until it has been tested for or when a cancer develops. According to the CDC, if we were to prevent Americans from contracting HPV, we would be preventing over 27,000 cases of cancer each year. When a gross estimate of the average cost to treat cancer is $150,000 per person, that would mean we would potentially save America over $4 billion annually.[17] Granted, that isn't enough to make a dent in our national deficit. Nevertheless, eradicating HPV would have significant cost-savings effects for Americans. It would prevent the loss of productivity from HPV-related cancer treatment and, of course, save lives.

The same is true for the hepatitis B virus (HBV), which is linked to liver cancer. HBV is spread via sexual contact as well as blood contact, and it's often found in intravenous drug users. Sadly, according to the CDC there are as many as 1.2 million people in the United States with this infection, and as with HPV, many are not aware they have it. Even more tragic, each year in the United States, up to 25,000 infants are born to mothers with HBV. Without intervention, 40 to 90 percent of these babies will become infected; approximately 90 percent of infected children develop chronic HBV infection. Early death from end-stage liver disease or liver cancer occur in over 25 percent of those with chronic HBV infection. Alcohol, obesity, and cryptogenic causes are the leading causes of chronic liver disease, but HBV infection is fourth in line for causing a cirrhotic liver, which costs roughly $35,000 to

$55,000 per patient annually to treat.[18] If we were able to prevent people from contracting hepatitis B infections, another 30,000 cancer deaths could be prevented, not to mention the tens of thousands of cases of chronic liver disease associated with the viral infection.

What if I told you there was a magic remedy that people could take to prevent HPV and HBV infections, and that insurance would even cover it without a co-pay—would you take it? Vaccinations to protect against both of these viruses are available, yet Americans have been slow to receive them. Australia is close to eradicating HPV infections because of its willingness to be proactive and vaccinate children and young adults against HPV. The United States has significantly lower levels of HPV vaccination rates. A related concern is the reemergence of measles, a virus once considered eradicated in America. That virus has made a comeback because of the irresponsible anti-vaccination, or "anti-vax," trend that runs rampant in the United States.

Catching Cancer Too Late

Let's say we change our habits, reduce our risk factors, and are successful at preventing many cancers. Still, we know that there are cancers we can't prevent. There are still things we can do to improve our outcomes after diagnosis. We can get screened to catch those cancers as early as possible. Cancer found in its later stages is harder to treat, and sometimes not treatable at all, bringing unnecessary suffering.

When breast cancer is detected with screening at an early stage, over 95 percent of women diagnosed will still be alive five years later, compared to only 15 percent of women diagnosed with the most advanced stage of disease. Similar numbers are seen for lung cancer, with more than 80 percent surviving for at least a year if diagnosed at the earliest stage compared to approximately 15 percent of those diagnosed with the most advanced stage of disease. Colon cancer has a 90 percent five-year survival rate if detected early with screening, versus a 14 percent five-year survival rate for late-stage diagnosis.[19]

Although estimates vary, the annual cost of cancer care in the United States is approximately $93 billion. In addition to saving or extending lives, prevention and early detection have the potential to reduce that financial burden through the reduction of treatment costs.

Most cancer research focuses on treatments for late-stage disease, with less than 15 percent of funding going toward early detection despite the fact that early intervention is far more effective at managing disease than late-stage therapy. A greater cost burden would be alleviated and more lives saved if we reoriented our approach to cancer care toward prevention and early detection.

Aside from prevention, the next step is education on disease symptoms to watch for and how to obtain cancer screenings. We need to improve public awareness of cancer symptoms and detection programs to encourage people to seek care when signs do arise. Most people are not aware that cancer often presents as a mild irritation.

A man repeatedly scratches a sore on his arm, thinking, "This thing won't go away." Lo and behold, it's skin cancer continuing to grow.

A woman finds that she's waking up in the middle of the night sweating and feeling sick. She feels tired during the day but assumes she's just sleep-deprived or needs a new mattress. But these can also be signs of leukemia and lymphoma.

A man notices blood in his stool, but it's just a little bit. Just a little bit can mean he has colon cancer. It can be cured if he goes to the doctor and it's found and treated right away. If he doesn't, it can kill him.

A woman notices that her nipple is inverting slightly, or it has a small area of dryness. She thinks it's probably nothing. But an underlying aggressive breast cancer may be there.

Similarly, irregular menstrual bleeding or spotting at odd times can mean uterine cancer. People with constant indigestion self-treat for an ulcer or "heartburn," when they may have gastric cancer or esophageal cancer. Sudden personality changes can mean brain cancer.

It's important to make clear that people should be aware of the symptoms to look out for and make an appointment with a doctor. We also need to invest in strengthening and incorporating health services and training for our health care workers, so they can conduct accurate and timely diagnostics. Ensuring access to cancer-screening programs like mammograms and colonoscopies is key. We also need to make sure people living with cancer receive effective treatment, including pain relief and social support services.

Challenges to accessing these services are significantly greater in low- and middle-income populations and in rural America, where there may be fewer physicians and radiology services available. Although rural America is seeing more accessibility through telemedicine programs and in-home services, its access to screening programs still needs improvement. If we want to decrease the overall cost burden of cancer for society, it is essential that we focus on early detection and treatment services in these vulnerable populations.

Dollars over People

As time has passed, our cancer treatments and detection methods have evolved. We've come a long way from the inception of cancer screening. The cancers we most commonly screen for are breast, cervical, colon, lung, and skin because these are the most common cancers and are cancers for which, when found early, the survival rates drastically increase as the overall cost of care decreases.

When a novel technology is introduced to the market, despite the testimony of physicians and patients as to how essential it is, insurance companies often do not want to cover the costs. Take breast cancer screening, for instance. For decades we used standard 2D mammography, which was shown time and time again to detect cancer earlier, yielding lower mortality rates from breast cancer. Better technology was then developed, including 3D mammography, whole-breast ultrasound, and MRI, which all improve cancer detection at the earliest stages. Yet medical professionals have to hire lawyers and billing experts to fight with the insurance companies to cover these updated (and improved) cancer detection modalities. I myself have spent countless hours talking to legislators and arguing with budget committees about the need to incorporate such technologies into covered cancer screenings. When insurance companies refuse to listen to reason, despite evidence of long-term cost savings, I feel we have no choice but to enlist the help of lawmakers. Asking the government to mandate coverage by private companies need not be in conflict with a belief in limited government and free markets. There are times when government regulation is required for the public good.

A major problem in US health care is the insurance industry's resistance to cover state-of-the-art cancer screenings. Ironically, insurance companies are a barrier to successfully detecting early, treatable cancers, which reduces costs for all. But if you think Canada's single-payer system is better at covering cancer screenings, it actually covers less than our system does.

The concept adopted by the insurers is why I didn't become an economist: insurers bet on you *not* developing cancer, but if you do, they will then cover treatments. I have a hard time wrapping my head around the notion of saving money up front by refusing to cover screenings, thereby leaving people to be diagnosed with late-stage cancers that will cost much more to treat—not to mention the increased suffering for the patient. Because of this unacceptable situation, I have helped lawmakers introduce and pass laws in Arizona, New Jersey, and New York to ensure that lower-income communities, and all women in general, have knowledge of and access to cancer-detection services. You wouldn't believe the fight I and my colleagues in this struggle had to put up just to make sure people had access to information about medical care.

Why did we have to enlist the legislative process to ensure that insurance will cover the use of the best cancer-detection technologies? Why couldn't we just say, "We have something that saves lives *and* will keep overall costs down—let's use it"? Unfortunately, insurers are gambling—with your life. So, perhaps now is the time to start taking back control.

Our Self-Imposed Cancer Paradox

The deductibles and co-pays that are features of most people's insurance plans are sometimes what keep people from getting the care they need. The Affordable Care Act eliminated the cost-sharing requirement for several cancer screenings, which increased screening utilization in some populations but had no effect on others. Despite aggressive efforts to increase breast (mammogram), colorectal (colonoscopy), cervical (Pap smears), and prostate (prostate-specific antigen [PSA] tests) cancer screenings over the past decade, screening rates remain suboptimal, with Americans not meeting the guidelines for recommended screenings.[20]

The guidelines for mammograms were updated in 2009 to recommend mammograms for women aged 50 to 75 every two years; the previous guidelines recommended mammograms for women 40 and older every one to two years. The guidelines for cervical cancer screenings were updated in 2012 to recommend a Pap smear for women aged 21 to 65 every three years; previously annual screenings were recommended for women who are sexually active. The ACA, which was passed in 2010, required more coverage by private insurance companies for these cancer screenings. However, the updated breast and cervical screening guidelines required fewer screenings and at longer intervals. The way I see it, these guidelines negatively affect younger women (40–49), who, when they get cancers, tend to have more aggressive cancers. This offsets the ACA's effort to cover care for more people.

Mandating insurance coverage and government subsidies to reduce the burden of cost sharing clearly isn't the answer. Rather, we need to remove other barriers to obtaining screenings by making the process easier—less time-consuming and less of a hassle. Part of the problem is that the system is overloaded with patients getting treated for preventable diseases. Insurance companies balk at covering preventative measures in part because they are shelling out billions of dollars a year on treatments for those illnesses.

As a nation we are stuck in a dichotomy: we want people to have earlier access to cancer detection, and we want the best methods to treat their cancer. Yet we are not focusing nearly enough on accountability for the self-destructive behaviors that drastically increase the chances of getting certain cancers and the issues that prevent us from getting screened. Eating poorly, not exercising, smoking, and failing to get recommended screenings all add to the high costs of health care in our great country and add to the burden of debt. We don't want to become a society in which those who don't engage in high-risk behaviors and who do follow screening guidelines get prompt, expert care, while those who don't take those precautions get delayed or subpar care. But to avoid such a scenario, we need to climb our way out of the mess we're in by doing two things: decreasing the cases of preventable cancers, and decreasing the cases of advanced cancers. If we can succeed at those goals, we will shift ample resources to the people who are suffering from cancers beyond anyone's control.

Chapter 5

INTO THE DEEP

America's Plunge into a Mental Health Epidemic

Americans are not only suffering physically but are confronting a growing mental health crisis that we are only beginning to understand. Mental health conditions are woefully undertreated in our country, largely because of the enduring stigma attached to mental illness. According to the National Institute of Mental Health, in 2017 only 42 percent of adults in the United States with a mental illness received mental health services.[1]

Although strides have been made over the past few decades in reducing the stigma, it's still easier to say "I have cancer" or "I have heart disease" than "I have bipolar disease" or "I have depression." Those coping with mental health problems may expect to encounter pity or condescension rather than the empathetic responses to physical diagnoses. People often keep mental health struggles private, or they fail to recognize them altogether.

We are all aware that, over our lifetimes, we have the risk of developing cancer, heart disease, or other illnesses. However, what is less known, or at least less acknowledged, is that we are also at risk for developing a mental disease. In any given year, approximately one in five adults in the United States experiences mental illness.[2] Take a look around you—it's much more likely that someone you know has some type of mental health disorder than, for example, a peanut allergy (only 5 percent of Americans, according to published data), yet think of how much awareness and caution are generated for that health issue.

You yourself may have some type of mental disorder and have yet to realize it. Anxiety disorders are the most common of all mental health issues and are on the rise. They affect just over 18 percent of the population. According to some mental health surveys, teens and young adults are more anxious than they've ever been before, and the trend is only strengthening. Half of all chronic mental illness begins by age fourteen and three-quarters by age twenty-four. Effective treatments are available, but according to the National Alliance on Mental Illness, there are long lags between the first appearance of symptoms and when people receive treatment, if they ever do.[3]

Whether or not people have empathy for those dealing with mental health problems, we need to pay attention to the impact of those problems on the country's financial burden. So here it is: setting aside the cost of treatment itself, America loses over $193 billion in earnings per year to serious mental illness when people are unable to work.[4] To make matters more alarming, those with a mental health disorder also face an increased risk of concurrent chronic medical conditions, such as obesity and heart disease. All of which drive up the cost of care for untreated mental illness.

Although we may try, it is impossible to separate mental from physical health. We urgently need to reshape our thinking about mental illness: we must look at it in the same way we view other health matters, with an eye to encouraging prevention where possible and treatment where needed. Only then can we prevent its costs—physical, mental, and financial—from overwhelming our capacities.

Complex Conditions

One reason for undertreatment of mental illness is misdiagnosis. This is an alarmingly common problem. Unfortunately, mental health disorders are not black and white—there are shades of gray that make diagnoses difficult. A mental health diagnosis cannot be easily confirmed with a single test, like a biopsy for cancer or a blood draw for an infection. Assessing a person for signs of mental illness requires particular expertise and finesse.

An obvious consequence of misdiagnosis is that it keeps people from receiving the treatment they need. The blunder of a misdiagnosis may allow anguish to grow, unchecked. With some types of disorders, this can potentially lead to destructive behaviors.

Let's pause and consider what we know about behavioral and emotional disorders. For the most part these afflictions cannot be diagnosed in a single visit to the doctor or from an imaging test. Rather, these diagnoses are based on clusters of reported feelings and behaviors that psychiatrists and psychologists must evaluate against standard definitions of a variety of mental disorders. Very often, there is a good deal of conjecture involved.

In patients coping with a mental disorder, normal life adaptability is often reduced. They may have trouble handling everyday problems and experience disruptions in normal thinking and behavior. They may feel like a round peg constantly being forced into the square hole of "normal" society. In order to avoid potentially disastrous outcomes, we must improve our ability to recognize the early signs of mental disorders and make treatment accessible.

For example, many of us may know a child or an adult who has fits of anger, sometimes spilling over into violence. You might simply call it a tantrum or having a bad day, but is it possible that they're suffering from something more serious that might be treatable? Often, disruptive behaviors will worsen over time, so ignoring them is not helpful to anyone.

Not everyone with a mental illness hallucinates or believes an alien invasion is imminent. In fact, most common mental health disorders are significantly more subtle. In order to understand the ways we can do better at treating mental health problems, it is essential to know more about the factors that cause them.

Varying Factors

There are many elements that contribute to the emergence and progression of mental health disorders. As with cardiovascular disease and cancer, biological factors we are born with play a role, as do social-environmental exposures we experience during our lives.

For some people, mental illness clusters in families, meaning it is part of their DNA. If there is a mutation or specific variant, this may make someone more susceptible to developing certain disorders. The most common disorders known to have some genetic component are autism, attention-deficit/hyperactivity disorder (ADHD), bipolar disorder, clinical depression (which differs from situational depression), and schizophrenia.

SITUATIONAL DEPRESSION VS. CLINICAL DEPRESSION

Situational depression is an occasional low mood due to certain circumstances (such as the death of a loved one or the loss of a job). Clinical depression has symptoms similar to those of situational depression, but they are severe enough to degrade a person's ability to maintain relationships, go to school or work, and perform everyday activities.

For conditions in which genes play a role, symptoms will usually appear by young adulthood. In many cases, the progression can be surprising. A child with a completely "normal" upbringing who has excelled, is the captain of the lacrosse team, and is a straight-A student might go off to college and suddenly begin dissociating from routine behaviors. His grades begin to slip. He isn't calling home much. When he comes home for a visit, he paces throughout the day, isn't sleeping well, and is just not his usual self. Maybe it's sleep deprivation, his parents think, or maybe even illicit drug use. But maybe it's something else. Just because the first eighteen years of his life he seemed as normal as any other kid doesn't mean he's healthy now. Whether the onset of mental disorders is brought on by the trauma of leaving home and being on one's own or is the timing of disease manifestation remains debatable.

It may take a major psychotic break, with delusions and/or hallucinations, or starkly erratic behaviors for the individual's family or friends to acknowledge that a mental illness is brewing. A psychotic episode does not equate to violence. Someone who is in a psychotic state may appear quite normal and have the same demeanor as always. However, there may be an underlying trigger that is waiting to be pulled.

My first lesson in this kind of situation happened while I was a young medical student on an inpatient psychiatric ward. It was at a county hospital that housed patients who had been institutionalized, prison inmates, and those with government insurance or none at all. Needless to say, it was extremely interesting to a student. After weeks of spending long days in the ward with patients, I became familiar with their behaviors and personalities. One of my favorite patients, Bob, had schizophrenia (manifested in disordered thinking and delusions) and spent most of his adult life in and out of institutions because of his inability to adapt to society. Or maybe it was our inability to adapt to him.

One day Bob was being interviewed by a pair of mental health workers for a new inpatient center across town. I was near enough to hear their conversation, which covered current events and philosophy. Bob was quite intelligent, and they saw little to suggest he qualified for their new facility, which was geared toward paranoid schizophrenics. As the interview began to wind down, I suspected that they were not convinced Bob would benefit from the new center. I walked over and slipped a note to one of the interviewers in which I had written, "Ask him about the glass." My note may have seemed odd, but sure enough Bob was asked about the glass. At that moment Bob's eyes narrowed and he began educating the interviewers on how the aliens had implanted glass under his skin to maintain control over his actions. All it took was a simple mention of his trigger to see the full extent of his disease. Had they not seen it, he would not have qualified for the treatment center. I often wonder about Bob and whether his mind failed or if we failed him. If we don't know how to bring out the thoughts deep within people like Bob, we are not recognizing the torment inside.

Unfortunately, when the torment goes unchecked, patients often require inpatient hospitalization to stabilize them. The most effective way to stabilize the severely mentally ill after a period of neglect is to give them heavy antipsychotic drugs in an attempt to help them regain a sense of reality.

Building Blocks of Mental Illness

Mental health disorders can be triggered by trauma or unsettling events in a person's life. When this happens, several afflictions can develop concurrently, such as depression, anxiety, and post-traumatic stress disorder (PTSD). Anyone can experience trauma— at home, in school, at work, or anywhere else in everyday life. Terrorist attacks and mass shootings have caused fear and anxiety throughout our society, but trauma is not limited to such violent events.

Veterans are a prime example of those at high risk for developing mental health disorders as a result of trauma. Military personnel consistently take care of their physical health during their arduous training and combat responsibilities but may neglect their mental and emotional health. In fact, according to a 2014 study, nearly one in four active-duty military personnel showed signs of a mental health condition.[5] Once they are back home, reacclimating to civilian life can cause anguish and feelings of isolation.

When our soldiers come home from active duty, they're often unable to recognize that they need mental health treatment. The ones who do recognize their need for help often stay silent, for fear of looking weak or perceived as a failure. For the minority of veterans who do turn to the Veterans Administration (VA) system for help, they can face long wait times—up to a year and a half to see a psychiatrist depending on which part of the country they live in.

We are doing a massive disservice to our veterans when we fail to provide them with the health care they need. Over one in ten homeless adults are veterans, and many homeless veterans suffer from PTSD and/or substance abuse disorders. These problems don't necessarily end when they find housing.[6]

A further critical issue concerning veterans is the suicide rate, which in 2016 was 1.5 times higher for veterans than for the rest of the adult population. From 2008 to 2016, there were over 6,000 suicides by veterans per year—a number that ought to shock us.[7] Suicide is always devastating, but when a person's suffering is a result of sacrifices made for our country, then every veteran suicide is an indictment on our society. This is especially true when veterans have tried to seek mental help only to be put on a wait list. Tragically, this happened to a friend of mine, a young man who had difficulty readjusting after a tour. He was not sleeping well and had nightmares. After months of pleading by his mother, he sought psychiatric help from the VA. He was given an appointment for an evaluation in six months, but killed himself in the interim. The VA system failed him. We need to do better—for our vets and for our country.

In general, we need to be more proactive in recognizing the signs of mental illness in ourselves and our loved ones. Left untreated, mental disorders can spiral out of control, and they can also lead people to self-medicate, which has even more detrimental consequences.

Self-Medication

Teens, young adults, and adults with mental illness tend to self-medicate with drugs (both legal and illegal), alcohol, and cigarettes to help ease their symptoms. The National Alliance on Mental Illness reports that over 44 percent of all cigarettes in the United States are consumed by adults with mental illness and/or substance abuse disorders.[8] As with the population as a whole, smoking puts people with mental illness at higher risk for major preventable diseases like heart disease, cancer, and lung disease.

Thinking back to when I was in residency, most inpatient psychiatric facilities had a smoking area. Many patients had fingers stained yellow from tobacco. I couldn't really understand why we were letting people smoke cigarettes. So I asked the attending psychiatrist, who told me, "You don't want to see them if they *can't* smoke," and then proceeded to explain how smoking affects their brain chemistry and symptoms. Especially if patients have schizophrenia or bipolar disorder, their paranoia is lessened by nicotine and alcohol. These drugs calm them and give them a euphoric feeling. Nicotine has mood-altering effects that can temporarily soothe the symptoms of mental illness, putting people with mental disease at significantly higher risk for nicotine addiction because they want that relief.

Mental illness also often leads to binge eating and unsafe sexual habits. Bipolar sufferers and schizophrenics especially tend to develop unsafe sexual practices. When they're manic, they may take part in a variety of risky behaviors they wouldn't ordinarily do, including unprotected sex with high-risk individuals, which may expose them to sexually transmitted diseases and unplanned pregnancies.

Sometimes teenagers with ADHD that goes untreated end up in the criminal justice system. Many of these children have trouble staying in school, and may lack a support structure at home. Of the 2 million youths arrested each year in the United States, up to 70 percent have a mental health disorder, according to the National Alliance on Mental Illness.[9]

People suffering from mental health disorders try to find relief in ways that, sadly, are harmful to their overall health and can be harmful to society. Steering people to the mental health support services they need is critically important.

Examining Diagnoses

As more people are being diagnosed with certain mental disorders, experts have considered whether there is an actual increase in the number of people with the disorder or only an increase in diagnoses. Anxiety disorders and depression, according to research, are indeed on the rise.[10] In the case of autism, increased awareness of this developmental disorder and changes in the criteria used to diagnose it have led to an increase in the number of diagnoses (not necessarily meaning that there are more people with autism).[11] When we hear about higher rates of one or another disorder, we want explanations. Some have jumped to blaming autism on vaccinations (which is simply wrong); others say social media and bullying are making us and our kids more anxious and depressed.

Although I think there is an arbitrarily increased prevalence of mental illness due to a lowered threshold of diagnostic criteria, we would be remiss to deny that our surroundings may be contributing to the increased incidence of such disorders.

THE SPECTRUM OF OBSESSIONS

Mental illness is not linear—it manifests on a spectrum. There are more than 200 recognized mental disorders. Some of the more common disorders are depression, bipolar disorder, dementia, schizophrenia, and anxiety disorders, with large variations in severity.

You can have very mild forms where you live your life without any kind of pharmacologic treatment; severe forms may require inpatient hospitalization and prevent a person from functioning independently. Most people live somewhere in between. For example, as a child I found myself constantly counting things—lines, shapes, objects. I'd count every square in my classroom, or certain features on people's faces. Despite my love of counting, it never disrupted my life. Surely my behavior was a mild form of obsessive-compulsive disorder (OCD).

Many people have focused thoughts or repeated behaviors like mine. But these thoughts do not disrupt their daily lives and may even make tasks easier. For this mildly abnormal behavior, no diagnosis or treatment is needed because it is not troublesome. For people with more serious OCD, thoughts stay agonizingly persistent, and unwanted repetitive behaviors interfere with normal daily activities and one's ability to function.

Like OCD, a mental disorder called body dysmorphic disorder (BDD) is linked to anxiety. The disorder usually surfaces in a person's teenage years and is characterized not only by obsessive thinking about a flaw in the sufferer's physical appearance, but by compulsive checking of the perceived defect (for example, ample time in front of the mirror), engaging in behaviors to minimize the appearance of the alleged flaw (such as excessive makeup, plastic surgery, social media filters), and hiding the disorder from others due to fear of social stigma.

In the era of social media, where it's easy to compare yourself unfavorably to others, we're feeding our anxieties, which is leading to a greater prevalence of OCD and BDD.

We live quickly and impulsively, demanding excellence from everyone. Bound to our desks at work and mesmerized by our smartphones during downtime, we're losing our sense of community and our place in social relationships. Furthermore, we are not getting the exercise or nutrition that our bodies and minds need.

Satisfying interpersonal relationships, whether with family, friends, or co-workers, lower the risk of depression and anxiety. Teens especially need personal relationships with their peer group, and social media friends don't necessarily count. For kids and adults alike, face-to-face interaction can reduce stress and fuel overall healthy development.

Technology and innovation have not only lessened our sense of community, but they have also heightened our desire for instant gratification. Don't get me wrong, I am on Facebook, Twitter, and Instagram. I don't know the intricacies like my children do, but I am plugged in nonetheless. We have yet to discover what long-term effects social media will have on our brains and functioning, not to mention our emotional well-being. But in the short term, we all see plenty of reasons to worry.

Our bodies are not built to withstand the barrage of information that we are constantly exposing ourselves to. A study in *Pediatrics* on babies who were exposed to television showed increased levels of cortisol (a stress hormone) when compared to babies who played with building blocks. A separate study in the same journal showed early television exposure significantly correlated with later diagnoses of ADHD. Fast-forward to all of the small children (including my own) I see in cars, restaurants, and airports with headsets and tablets playing games and watching videos. Yes, adults need a break sometimes from entertaining their kids, but we may be lessening our own stress hormones while raising our children's. Ultimately, we may be raising children to have a lower threshold for stress and anxiety.

In the digital age, instant gratification is the way we live now.

No more family debates around the dinner table—as soon as a disagreement arises, the nearest piece of technology is consulted to prove someone right or wrong. No more counting games or staring out the window on long road trips—kids just watch videos. Forget about moments of uncomfortable silence in a conversation, when both parties need to navigate out of the awkwardness—we're staring down at our phones instead of having conversations.

We don't use cash any more, we swipe a credit card. We don't go into restaurants to wait for our takeout food to be prepared, we use the drive-through or a digital app for ordering. Newspapers are an antiquity because of Twitter feeds and digital alerts. Many of us don't even buy our own groceries anymore, we have them delivered. How easy do we need to make things for ourselves? Should we not do anything on our own? Are we relying so much on technology and placing such a high value on convenience that we are losing our coping mechanisms when something unexpected or even slightly stressful occurs?

The need for the latest and greatest technologies has even made its way into health care. Patients get their blood drawn, leave the hospital, then later that day log in to their patient portal online to see their lab results. The doctors haven't interpreted the lab findings, but the patients want the results now. When a CT scan is ordered, the patient requests the report directly without even consulting the ordering doctor to help interpret the findings of the scan. This begs the question, should everyone have access to their health information? Of course they should. In fact, the surprising driver of health care technology innovation today is largely created by impatience and the need to deliver.

Yet how much of our anxiety is a result of our unwillingness to slow down and wait for things?

DON'T LET ANXIETY BE AN EXCUSE

We seem to use the words "stress" and "anxiety" interchangeably these days. They do share many of the same physical symptoms, but an anxiety disorder is quite different from anxiety/stress.

Stress is often a normal reaction to situations and usually not a medical condition requiring treatment. At other times, however, we can develop anxiety without a triggering event, and it can be a sustained state. Usually short-term, stress is our body kicking into gear when we need it to (to meet a deadline, give a speech, take a test, get ourselves out of danger, etc.). Negative stress, on the other hand, is when the body has a negative reaction to something (such as when we can't sleep or have impaired concentration). But again, it can be normal to have these negative responses depending on the situation. An anxiety disorder tends to be long-term rather than situational and can affect a person's relationships, ability to work, and so on. Different from a mild or vague unsettling feeling, an anxiety disorder can prevent a person from functioning.

While it is true that we are finding ourselves exposed to more situations that lead to mental health disorders, it appears more people are in fact being diagnosed with anxiety because we're putting more behaviors and feelings under the anxiety "umbrella." Because of our expanded definition of anxiety, we may be overmedicating some people as a quick fix to get them back to feeling good. Our overdiagnosis and -treatment of perceived disorders are making Americans too sensitive to their environments, and their diagnoses are potentially functioning as a crutch. When we are feeling stressed, simple steps like counting to ten or taking deep breaths might be all we need to get through it. Working on behavioral and lifestyle changes to reduce or cope with stress may eliminate the need to take a pill. With the increased diagnosis of anxiety, we are taking away from the gravity of true anxiety disorders and the anguish they can cause.

Younger people are using anxiety as an excuse for their perceived problems. This may explain the call for "safe spaces" and "mental health days" on college campuses. In 2019, Oregon passed a law that requires high schools to allow up to five absences every three months to be used as mental health days, in addition to absences allowed for being sick. Is this setting kids up for failure once they hit the real world, where most employers expect their employees to show up for work?

The Price of Perfection

In 2016 the National College Health Assessment discovered a frightening but largely underreported phenomenon: nearly 63 percent of all college students reported feeling "overwhelming anxiety" within the last year. That's a 50 percent increase from just five years earlier. The United States has a higher incidence of anxiety than the rest of the world, where the global prevalence of anxiety is about 7 percent. As a whole we are more anxious and it seems we aren't doing much to stave it off in our youth. Adolescents and young adults in the United States have not only become more anxious over the last few decades, but they represent the most anxious age group among all Americans. Moreover, they are more anxious than their peers across the rest of the world.[12]

What is going on in America in the twenty-first century to make the younger generation anxious? Setting aside the fact that there is some level of overdiagnosis, I believe we are creating a toxic culture for our children.

Comparing Ourselves to Death

According to a report on two surveys of adolescents, published in the journal *Clinical Psychological Science*, during the period 2010–2015 the number of thirteen- to eighteen-year-olds who had symptoms of depression went up by 33 percent, and the number who committed suicide increased by 31 percent. The same study found that teens who spent more time on social media were more likely to describe themselves as having mental health issues than those who spent more time on other activities.[13]

Now we have researchers exploring how "digital addiction," like any other form of addiction, leads to higher levels of feeling isolated, depressed, and anxious.[14] The supermodels and fitness experts flaunting their bodies on social media are enough to make anyone feel inadequate, let alone an impressionable teenager. While social media does provide a place for discussion, venting, support, and advice, if everyone is commiserating, is that really helpful? Looking through social media feeds proves that digital misery may, in fact, love digital company.

Chasing Perfection

Then there are the celebrities of social media like the Kardashians— the royal family of digital white noise. I know I have already mentioned this family, but they are such an apt example of the points

I'm making, how could I not return to them? In the era of reality TV, this is how people are making their fortunes: simply by living their vapid lives in front of a camera. The Kardashians and their entourage embark on private jets and wear custom-made designer clothes for which they often pay nothing because they are the perfect marketing tool. It is comical that the people who have an abundance of money are most likely receiving much of their gear gratis. Then comes the sad spectacle of everyone else trying to imitate them without the same financial means.

Bravo to those who have become wealthy and are living the life of luxury. The majority of Americans, though, probably don't make as much as the Kardashians' housekeepers, so trying to emulate them via social media is folly.

It is anything but funny when people go broke trying to mimic celebrities. For example, a twenty-six-year-old woman named Lissette Calveiro nearly went bankrupt trying to become an Instagram star. She posted pictures of herself online doing exotic poses in foreign lands. She blogged about all her travels with accompanying photograms. Unfortunately, she didn't have the funds to support such a lavish lifestyle. Lissa moved to New York for an internship in 2013, and she felt like she was living the *Sex and the City* dream. However, she wound up going into massive debt. She spent money she didn't have on jet-setting travel, attending high-end brunches, and wearing designer clothing, all to impress her social media followers.

Her internship provided only a small stipend, so she worked part-time at a retail store to supplement her income. I must applaud her industriousness, but her focus was off-target. She squandered her income in a quest to portray the "perfect" lifestyle. Her goal had been to tell her story as a young millennial living in New York City. Instead, she racked up about $10,000 worth of debt while living a life she could not actually afford. She was a young millennial trying to keep up with social pressures.

The wannabe celebrity lifestyle not only has financial consequences but is conducive to body dysmorphic disorder and a new form of anxiety. Making a social media post "like-worthy" isn't just about having a perfect smile—there must also be the perfect outfit, the perfect background, the perfect makeup, and, let's not forget, the perfect digital touch-ups. Yet even with a perfect post, rejection can ensue. Striving for social media stardom can bring on a barrage of negative comments. Even the simple fact of a follower not acknowledging a post can feel like rejection.

For so many young people, this lack of desired attention online equates to not being a part of the "cool crowd" in high school or being the last one chosen for the kickball team. This social rejection can cause a person's sense of self-worth to spiral downward, even when the person outwardly projects the picture-perfect life.

As a direct side effect of our culture's demand for Hollywood-level perfection, young people are modifying their bodies more than ever. This "perfection" is not being sought through hard work and determination but through quick fixes. Parents are giving kids breast augmentation surgeries for their high school graduation. Teens get Botox injections so easily you'd think they were vitamins rather than toxins. We're allowing our children to alter their appearance before they've even had a chance to accept who they are. A young girl who has a complex about her lips often has other underlying insecurities that are hidden because her self-consciousness is manifesting as an obsessive desire to "fix" a single body part. Perhaps she's a little overweight, has normal hormonal acne, or felt rejection at school because the boy she liked did not pay attention to her. If she believes changing one aspect of her appearance will improve her life, she will be deeply disappointed when she learns it doesn't. And that begins the domino effect of anxiety and the quest to find physical perfection. There will always be more that can be "enhanced" on our bodies. The earlier we begin altering our physical appearance to satisfy our mental health, the more we will do so throughout our lifetimes and the less work we will be doing on our inner (and outer) selves.

I want to be clear that not everyone who gets cosmetic surgery has body dysmorphic disorder. In fact, the majority of people who have plastic surgery do not suffer from it. However, it is increasingly troublesome to watch a generation of children who look at the body God gave them and see it as nothing more than a suggestion.

Before you start having needles stuck in yourself or your child, pursue the optimal natural version of yourself, mentally and physically. Exercise, eat right, and spend quality time with your family and friends to achieve an overall sense of wellness.

Get yourself to your true best. If at that point you still want something done surgically, then go for it. Don't just jump into an expensive medical procedure without making the effort yourself, and please stop allowing your children to do that. Fixing our appearance will do nothing for us if we don't work to stave off preventable diseases like cardiovascular disease and cancer, and if we don't take care of our mental health. In fact, it may worsen anxiety and depression. If we aren't equally focusing inward, then our efforts at outer self-improvement are futile.

Schoolhouse Blues

The oldest of my three children grew up in classrooms dominated by the No Child Left Behind Act. This bipartisan federal legislation, signed into law by President George W. Bush in 2002, mandated standardized testing in every public school in America. Because of this requirement, we have kindergartners taking timed tests on reading and writing, instead of focusing on crafts, physical activity, and socialization skills. Children are preparing for the anticipated exams from the moment they walk in the door.

By high school, high-achieving students face overwhelming pressure to succeed. Their parents often place high expectations on them, leaving them feeling stressed, inadequate, apprehensive, and depressed. Obsessing over which college they get into has eaten up their lives along with their parents' lives. Isn't it more important for our children to grow up feeling confident and content than to get accepted to a school we, as their parents, want them to attend? Why do we pressure them like this? We tell ourselves we want what is best for our children, but we fall prey to the same social acceptance pressures our children do. As adults, aren't we also trying to impress our colleagues or climb the ladder of social status based on our children's accomplishments? Where our children go to school has become a status symbol for adults, as though we should be commended for *their* achievements.

For kids who are already perfectionists, this stress to excel only exacerbates their worries. When they get the first B of their lives, they worry it will prevent them from going to college—not just their dream college but any college. On top of that, they don't want to disappoint us, their parents. Our unreasonable expectations for our children are hurting them, both physically and mentally. Who are we really serving—our children or ourselves? The answer is neither.

When the Stress Is Too Much

It was my son's senior year of high school, and admissions letters were streaming into everyone's inbox. An acquaintance of my son had applied to his father's alma mater; it had been ingrained in him since he was young that he would go to that school. He'd been active in sports and did well academically, in hopes of fulfilling his father's dream. But ultimately, he received a rejection letter.

After he read the decision, he wrote his own letter to his family, left it on the kitchen table, took his father's gun with him as he drove to his local church, and killed himself.

An overwhelming sympathy for the devastation his parents felt consumed my heart. As the mother of three boys, I found it even more distressing to imagine the immense desperation that young boy felt as he sat there in the pew of his hometown church. Moments before he pulled the trigger, what was he feeling? Did he feel anything at all, or was he lost in a darkness of self-perceived failure and despair? The thought of any person ever feeling that their life is not worth living, the utter anguish of it, is heartbreaking. That, to me, is more devastating than any diagnosis I have ever given.

Mental illness can cause long-term effects and suffering. Like my son's classmate, children are dying as a result. Those with mental illness, even the mildest forms of depression, have an increased risk of suicide, and the risk is increasing among our children.

Think about these statistics: Suicide is the second-leading cause of death among teenagers aged fifteen to nineteen, and the third-leading cause of death in all children under fifteen.[15]

At a time when their bodies are still healthy and their responsibilities limited, when everything is possible, they're taking their own lives.

As parents, we try to instill in our children a striving for success and accomplishment. We think we are encouraging them to be the best they can be, and often we are. But occasionally our expectations have the opposite effect. Was the demand to get into his father's college so oppressive as to drive the boy to take his own life, or were the circumstances misunderstood? I know nothing of the family's dynamics, but I know there is no college in the world worth a child's life, and I am certain his parents would agree with me.

As grown-ups, we are creating circumstances that leave our children feeling abandoned and fragmented. Our high expectations for them, both at home and in school, with the emphasis on standardized testing, come from our desire to give them the best lives possible. However, the pressures we put on them are leading to anxiety, depression, and, yes, even suicide. For centuries, successful men and women have worked their way to the top on their own volition. In the last several years my generation has coined the term "helicopter parents" because we are always hovering over our kids. This phenomenon can be seen in the recent college admissions scandal involving Hollywood celebrities and other wealthy parents paying hundreds of thousands of dollars to get their children into prestigious schools on the basis of falsified test scores and made-up athletic achievements. By clearing the obstacles in our children's path, some of us are surely going too far in our role as parents.

Given how recently the concept entered the culture, only a few small-scale studies have explored the effects of helicopter parenting. Not surprisingly, these studies show that overparenting, especially of late teens, breeds narcissism and poor coping skills. Often the traits produced by this type of parenting are associated with amplified stress and anxiety in the children (parents too).

Happy and healthy—this is what I want my children to be. In my parenting routine, I encourage a healthy diet and ample physical activity. I make sure my kids get the recommended vaccinations, and I teach them to use sunscreen when needed. As I read articles about parenting, I realize I too am guilty of many of the behaviors that meet the criteria for helicoptering. Rather than rationalizing our parental intrusions, for whatever reason, what if we step back a bit and see what the kids can do without our intervention? Or rather, what they *want* to do. Perhaps if we loosened the reins on children and allowed them to thrive in their own way we might lessen the risk of mental health disorders and suicide in our youth. The first step is acknowledging there is a problem rather than ignoring the truth.

#MentalHealthMatters

I cannot harp enough on the truth that it is imperative to give mental health the attention it deserves. Suicide has continued to rise steadily since 1999, and according to the CDC, more than half of all people who commit suicide have no known mental health condition. What I see in that statistic is that nearly half of people who kill themselves *are* suffering from a mental health disorder, whether a mild case of situational depression or severe schizophrenia. Excluding the outliers that may be attributable to the hardships of the financial crisis during this time, I would hazard a guess that the remaining suicides were driven by undiagnosed mental health conditions.

Across the country, people are joining the #MeToo and #TimesUp movements. Sexual assault and gender discrimination have stayed under the radar and it was time for a change. Inappropriate behavior is being called out, and we are seeing mountains being moved. I would say it is time for a similar mental health awareness movement. We need to make sure mental health gets the attention necessary to spur action. Now that legislators and even the president are using social media as a political forum, perhaps a hashtag would make this happen. With enough momentum, it would certainly raise eyebrows, and I am confident legislators would take notice.

Attention by legislators could translate into health policy geared toward helping Americans dealing with mental health disorders. For a start, mental health should be covered by insurance at the same level as physical health. The Affordable Care Act began integrating the two, but we have much further to go. Psychiatrists are grossly underrepresented in the medical community, and that's because our country prioritizes other specialties. Until depression or bipolar disorder is seen the way doctors view rheumatoid arthritis or a brain tumor diagnosis, mental illness won't get the support it needs.

Anxiety and depression can sneak up on you if you're not careful. We aren't watching closely enough for the signs of mental instability—until it's too late. After each mass shooting, mental health gets a brief moment in the spotlight only to fade quickly. We shouldn't be waiting for a suicide, a mass shooting, or an addiction to concern ourselves with mental health. Let's start right now by taking practical steps, whether it's wellness activities or making ourselves more aware of those around us. Let's resolve to remove the stigma from mental illness. That's the only way we'll ensure a future of mental and emotional well-being for ourselves and for others. Let's start a new movement, drawing inspiration from the See Something, Say Something antiterrorism campaign: If you see someone who may need help with a mental health problem, say something before it's too late.

Chapter 6

THE OPIOID CRISIS

Mental health problems and substance abuse go hand in hand. As American deaths from suicide and drug overdoses hit an all-time high, it is important to highlight the fact that opioids are responsible for six out of every ten overdose deaths in the United States. This nationwide crisis of opioid use has been brewing for a while. Before we can figure out how to fix it, we need to understand how it began. It should come as no surprise that the opioid crisis finds its origins in our need for instant gratification. In order to begin to address this calamity, let us identify the players and the role of American impulsivity.

Using opiates, natural substances derived from the opium poppy, to treat pain is an ancient practice. In 460 BC, Hippocrates, known as the father of medicine, used white poppy juice to alleviate various ailments. In 1806, a German chemist named Friedrich Sertürner isolated morphine from opium and named it after Morpheus, the Greek god of dreams.

Throughout the nineteenth century, morphine was a mainstay of medical treatment in the United States, treating a variety of afflictions from pain to respiratory problems and even anxiety.

During the Civil War, opiates were used for pain control and palliation. Many soldiers treated with morphine for their injuries became addicted to it. In fact, after the war, morphine addiction was known as "soldier's disease" and became normalized in the eyes of the public. In the early 1900s, heroin, another opiate, was believed to be a nonaddictive alternative to morphine and was introduced as a painkiller. The Saint James Society, a philanthropic group, mailed free samples of heroin to morphine addicts, thinking it would help cure them of their addiction. That, of course, was a terrible idea.

Heroin sales eventually stopped with the passage of the Heroin Act of 1924, making the possession and manufacturing of heroin illegal. In a dramatic effort to stave off the crisis of addiction, the Heroin Act even made the medicinal use of heroin illegal. Physicians were outraged because opiates were considered a useful tool in the medical community, with many physicians using them to treat pain, alcoholism, and other addictions.

In the 1960s and 1970s, during the Vietnam War, illegal heroin was smuggled into the United States from Southeast Asia, an area that is a major producer of opium. In 1969 the World Health Organization (WHO) took the position that the medical use of morphine did not lead to dependence. WHO clarified this position by stating that tolerance and physical dependence do not constitute a drug addiction, thus suggesting that there was a mental component to addiction separate from the physical effects. Simply because the *body* is addicted to something, according to that view, doesn't mean that the *person* is mentally addicted. The complexity of addiction to opiates was essentially reduced to the simplistic concept of mind over matter. Unfortunately, WHO failed to recognize that physical dependence and mental addiction are in fact entangled—it's difficult to have one without the other. Addiction is even more difficult to treat if these two aspects are viewed as separate phenomena.

An estimated half million Americans became hooked on heroin. By the mid-1980s heroin use decreased again as more people began using crack cocaine. During the crack epidemic, four or five million Americans became addicted. Since the attention was diverted momentarily from opiates, in the mid-1970s synthetic versions of opiates called "opioids" began production, including fentanyl. In the 1990s physicians began prescribing opioid pain-killers more frequently, as they were assured by pharmaceutical companies that these drugs were not addictive. Purdue Pharma, a pharmaceutical company owned by the Sackler family, became the megaproducer of the now infamous OxyContin, a drug that hit the market in 1996.

In 2001 the Joint Commission on Accreditation of Healthcare Organizations (JCAHO) put forth new standards for pain management. Now called simply the Joint Commission, this organization is a self-appointed group of administrators that surveys hospitals with innumerable checklists ostensibly to ensure that proper care is being provided. Would it be going too far to compare this intrusive group of health care bureaucratic intruders to the wise guys who routinely stop by the bodega to make sure things are in line but do not provide any benefit to the overall function of the bodega? It depends on which side of the Joint Commission line you sit on, I suppose.

The Joint Commission expected everyone to comply with its new standards, effective immediately. They named pain the "fifth vital sign." This is when charts showing ten faces ranging from smiling to grimacing began to appear in emergency rooms and doctors' offices to help patients rate their pain from 1 to 10. Physician groups were outraged and advocated against it. They acknowledged that we must provide patients with pain control but argued that pain is not a vital sign, which is a clinical measurement (e.g., blood pressure, heart rate, temperature, respiratory rate). Physicians were concerned about the ramifications of constantly chasing pain. The choice of a face to express the extent of pain being experienced is not clinically measurable.

In addition to this new pain chart, the Centers for Medicare and Medicaid Services (CMS; the federal agency in charge of administering government health insurance programs) began emphasizing patient satisfaction surveys on pain control as part of its reimbursement procedures. The goals of the pain chart and satisfaction surveys were to help patients communicate, and doctors to alleviate, pain; but they also became a constant reminder to the doctor of the need to make certain that pain was managed to a level satisfactory to the patient. The question is, how do you decide what pain levels are acceptable? If someone had a recent surgery, should we expect them to be in no pain? Because of these new requirements imposed from outside the medical community, physicians were no longer able to make decisions on the level of appropriateness of patients' pain. Instead, they had to focus on the customer-service side of pain control—all of this to ensure proper compensation for their services rendered. With the heavy-hitting pharmaceutical companies aggressively marketing inexpensive and effective pain medication to physicians with limited pain management education, it's no wonder their use skyrocketed. One thing the pharmaceutical companies knew but physicians didn't was that opioid tablets, once crushed or dissolved, could be snorted, smoked, or injected, making it easy to abuse them.

We Should Have Seen It Coming

As soon as that fifth vital sign was introduced, more opioid prescriptions were written, and Big Pharma jumped all over it. They continued pushing their products and producing variant opioids. They told physicians each new formulation was less addictive, when really they'd just made longer-acting pills that were harder to crush. This did nothing to thwart the crisis we are now in; rather, it just increased their profits. In the early 2000s, reports of abuse were well known, and in 2003 the Drug Enforcement Agency (DEA) found that the aggressive marketing methods used by Purdue Pharma had "very much exacerbated OxyContin's widespread abuse."

Doctors were overprescribing opioids, and most didn't even know it. Until recently, medical schools offered minimal, if any, education in pain management and even less in addiction treatment. Pharmaceutical companies knew this, and as revealed by whistleblowers, they targeted primary-care doctors with their marketing schemes for entry-level opioids. The highly skilled sales representatives were shoving their self-funded rubbish studies down doctors' throats, saying everything was fine and there was minimal risk of addiction. They even suggested that the only people who became addicted to prescription opioids were the people who are drug addicts already. Why would physicians believe anything different with a lack of education to disprove these claims? It was less than a few decades earlier that WHO told us something similar regarding addiction, that it was mostly in the head and could be controlled if an addict wanted to. The culmination of mistakes doctors made as a result of these misgivings had devastating consequences.

OPIOID ABUSE STATS

The abuse of opioids significantly increased in the early to mid-2000s, nearly doubling between 1998 and 2009 as a result of the increased prescribing of these drugs for pain. An estimated 4 to 6 percent who misuse prescription opioids transition to heroin. About 80 percent of people who use heroin first misused prescription opioids. Deaths from prescription opioids more than quadrupled from 1999 to 2016, with more than 63,000 Americans dying from opioid overdose in 2016.[1]

Today, on average, $20 billion is spent on hospital care for opioid overdoses every year in the United States.

No One Is Immune

Without a doubt, the opioid crisis has affected all parts of America, across all socioeconomic groups and regions. In a national poll released by the American Psychiatric Association in 2018, one in three Americans said they know someone addicted to opioids, and more than half of millennials said they think getting illegal opioids is easy.[2]

No one is immune to this devastation when over 2 million Americans were classified as misusing prescription pain relievers in 2017 alone.[3] From our homeless populations to college students to unemployed factory workers to stay-at-home moms, anyone can become addicted.

Think of this scenario: Sally was home alone one day with her kids off to school and her husband away. She decided to replace a lightbulb in the living room ceiling fixture, which required a stepladder to reach. Her flimsy slipper got caught on the top step, and she fell a few feet to the ground. It wasn't that traumatic a fall but it was enough to break a bone and require a trip to the ER. At the ER, they confirmed with an x-ray a broken bone in her wrist and put her in a cast, also giving her ten days' worth of opioids to manage the pain. Sally didn't know then what we now have proved to be true. After three days of consuming opioids there's a significantly higher chance of becoming addicted. Chances are the doctor who wrote the prescription didn't know, either. So, following doctor's orders, she took them for all ten days, and when she finished the supply her body began to tell her she needed more.

She calls her doctor, and he believes her wrist could still be giving her pain—after all, it's broken and she is home taking care of three small children. So now she gets another five days' worth of opioids. She doesn't fit the profile of a patient at high risk of addiction. She just needs more pain control to allow her arm to heal. At the end of that prescription, she calls the doctor back. This time, he declines to fill another prescription. But her body is dependent on the pills at this point, and is telling her it needs more. So, she can go see another doctor about it. If she's really desperate, she might even take off her wrist brace and go to an urgent care complaining of an injured wrist. They will do an x-ray to see if it's broken and, lo and behold, she has a broken wrist. They'll treat her for her broken wrist just the same as the ER did. The opioid addiction cycle has begun. When the legal prescriptions run out, Sally will try to find alternate sources for her pills. She might even turn to heroin use.

This may sound outlandish to some, but let me assure you, this is common all across America. According to the National Institute on Drug Abuse, 86 percent of heroin users initially used opioid pain relievers, which is markedly different from the 1960s, when over 80 percent of abusers started with heroin.[4]

Now let me tell you about a real story of addiction. When I was growing up in Arizona, one of my favorite pastimes was horseback riding. On a warm, late-spring morning, my mom and I went out to the desert for a quick ride. For whatever reason, on a seemingly perfect day my mom's horse got spooked. He bucked up on his hind legs and threw my mom off. She landed awkwardly with her arms stretched out forward. Immediately we could see the deformity of her left wrist. It was indented, like a cartoon character who's been hit in the arm with a rod. She immediately went into shock from the pain and fear. With the sun beating down, I propped her on my horse and we sped back to the house. We hurriedly jumped in the car and headed to the hospital.

She was in surgery almost immediately to repair broken bones and injured tendons and nerves. Her wrist was fastened internally with metal plates and screws, and she was told that, without aggressive physical therapy, the nerve damage would likely be permanent. Upon her release, she was prescribed OxyContin not only for the acute pain following surgery but for the pain she would endure during stringent physical therapy and from continued neuropathic pain from the damaged nerves. The medication came as extended-release tablets, and taking two or three a day hardly felt excessive. She continued the prescribed regimen for many months during therapy and healing. It wasn't until her own mother, my grandmother, fell gravely ill that things started to unravel. Because she would be flying to New York to spend time with her mother and not continuing physical therapy, my mom did not fill her last prescription. Without the OxyContin, she flew to New York to care for her mother.

At that point, her body was dependent on the daily dose of opioids, but she had no idea. Within twenty-four hours of departing for New York, she became violently ill. Although she had classic symptoms of opioid withdrawal, she had no idea what was wrong. She believed she had contracted a terrible illness, with diarrhea, vomiting, anxiety, severe abdominal cramping, fast heart rate, tremor, and muscle pain. Instead of being by her ailing mother's bedside, she herself was fighting for her life and had to be hospitalized.

Thankfully, the doctors and staff were astute enough with their history-taking and medical management that they safely stabilized her. They explained to her it had been the lack of opioids that made her so violently ill. When she now recounts this story, she says it was as though she had lost control of her body. She truly felt as though she were going to die.

My mother was lucky. Although it may not seem that way with all she went through, the truth is many others experience brutal withdrawal symptoms in a nonmedical setting and urgently re-supply their body with opioids to avoid them. It may have been her initial ignorance of the early symptoms of withdrawal that saved her from a future of addiction. She sought medical attention be-cause she thought an infection was wreaking havoc in her body. Had she known her symptoms could be stopped by consuming pain medication, the outcome may have been very different. My mother is not an addict, but the fear of addiction stigma is strong in everyone, and avoidance is an easy out.

As we are recognizing the abuse potential of these powerful medications, many physicians have voluntarily limited the amount they prescribe; they may even give patients drug tests to help mon-itor for abuse. At some point, the well does run dry and patients can no longer obtain legally prescribed opioids. Based on the level of physical dependence, people may do anything they can to avoid withdrawing—whether that's going through the medicine cabinet at their parents' and friends' houses to see if they have any unused bottles of pills, to eventually obtaining it illegally on the streets.

Not all illegal drug deals are in back alleys, as in the movies. Opioids are much more accessible than anyone wants to believe. At work. In our schools. Everywhere. We think to ourselves, "I don't even know how I would obtain heroin." But let me tell you something as an experienced physician: when you're addicted, you will find it. These drugs are much more prevalent and available than you can imagine.

Baby Steps Forward

In 2016, as the opioid crisis was running rampant, the American Medical Association finally removed pain as a fifth vital sign. According to the American Society of Addiction Medicine (ASAM), by that point over 300 million opioid prescriptions had been written, more than enough to give a bottle to every American adult.[5] Better late than never, I suppose. Many movements since have been implemented across the nation to monitor prescription trends and limit use. In 2017, the Trump administration began aggressively tackling the crisis by distributing the first round of a $485 million grant to the fifty states and US territories to help combat opioid abuse. In the same year, then Attorney General Jeff Sessions launched the Opioid Fraud and Abuse Detection Unit within the Department of Justice, with a mission to prosecute individuals who commit opioid-related health care fraud.[6] In 2018, President Trump signed the SUPPORT for Patient and Communities Act, expanding access to treatment for substance use disorders and promoting research for nonaddictive pain management methods. Data available in early 2020 reported that US opioid deaths decreased in 2018, after years of steady increases.

Where Do We Go from Here?

Since we recognize over 80 percent of people who are addicted to opioids started out on legally prescribed opioid medications, what do we do going forward? Law enforcement is solely one part of a bigger picture. For example, police can't control when teenagers and young adults obtain pills from their parents' and grandparents' medicine cabinets. The same poll from ASAM told us teenagers share or sell their unused prescription pain medications (prescribed for wisdom teeth removal, orthopedic injuries, etc.) to their friends or relatives. No amount of increased police presence or border security will prevent that.

Clearly we also need to decrease the number of legal opioids available so they don't get in the wrong hands. For that, we can implement pharmaceutical buy-back programs, which would work like this: if you have pills left from your prescription, stop keeping the bottles in your medicine cabinet and bring them back to the pharmacy. There should be incentives, such as $5 off your next prescription, to do this. Many police stations have set up drop-off centers, where you can drop unused pills in a locked box. These drop boxes are underused, however, and incentives from the pharmacy are likely to work better.

We could also shorten the duration of the prescriptions when possible. If someone breaks a bone, we know they likely will need only three days' worth of opioids, and that's all they should be prescribed. Instead of a universal restriction on all opioid pre-scriptions, we can shorten the length for particular ailments. Also, a centralized system to monitor who is receiving opioids is essential to eliminate "doctor shopping" and overuse of medications. How-ever, even as I declare support for some of these endeavors, I know the key is to stop generalizing about those suffering because pain is certainly not one size fits all.

The urgency to "fix" the problem has prompted well-meaning but uninformed legislators to introduce laws that place restrictions on prescribing doctors. In addition to the government, insurance companies and even pharmacies are limiting the number of days or quantities for which physicians can prescribe opioids; this approach has its merits, but it also has a negative impact on chronic pain patients. Acute pain experiences from an injury or after surgery may require only a few days of medication, but what about patients with chronic pain, those suffering from agonizing pain related to cancer, or veterans who cope with lingering pain from traumatic limb amputations? Until you have sat with a man who has lost his legs from an IED blast overseas and now lives with intolerable phantom pain that is relieved only by opioids, or the elderly woman in a nursing home whose bones are breaking every day because of advanced cancer, you cannot talk to me about who should or should not have the authority to dole out pain medication. I have sat with both of these patients and know there *is* still medicinal use for opioids. By blindly restricting a doctor's prescription rights, we're also limiting opioid access for the patients that legitimately need relief.

Centralization is a great way to communicate and lessen overprescribing, but these systems are expensive, with most of the cost placed on the physician. Various states are working on a streamlined system so that Dr. A is aware that Dr. B prescribed an opioid for a patient, to vastly reduce the amount of "doctor shopping" that addicts often resort to.

In addition to limiting legally prescribed opioids, while ensuring patients with pain are still adequately treated, we also need to make illegal forms of opioids unobtainable. These drugs have been flooding into our nation from China; they are also carried across our southern and northern borders. How can anyone deny that we need effective border control in the midst of an opioid epidemic? Without strong borders, opioids and other illicit drugs will continue to flood our streets, and our neighbors will keep overdosing and dying. We must deal more harshly with those who are bringing illegal drugs from outside the country and those who are supplying it from within our borders. The prescription restrictions and mental health awareness efforts are futile if we can't rid our neighborhoods of illegal opioids.

Those addicted to opioids suffer from the stigma that they "did it to themselves," which prompts questions about whether the government is obligated to fund efforts to counteract a self-inflicted crisis. Does the same hold true for those with lung cancer from smoking, high cholesterol from a poor diet, or back pain from being overweight? Do we get to judge someone for a drug addiction but not others whose lifestyle choices led to preventable conditions and diseases? As a society, we struggle with our attitude toward people with addiction, and with how much responsibility we expect addicts to take for their problem. Each addiction may be the individual's problem, but the opioid crisis is collectively all our problem.

Another thought is whether addicts who use illicit drugs belong behind bars. It can be argued that addiction itself is punishment enough. Also, wouldn't it better our country to have them back as functioning members of society rather than adding to the prison population? Numerous studies found that placing criminal offenders with a history of drug and alcohol abuse in addiction treatment programs would not only cut crime rates but save billions of dollars from negating loss productivity.[7]

In 2018, President Trump signed the First Step Act, a criminal justice reform bill aimed at reforming many of the tough-on-crime federal policies of the 1980s and 1990s. This was a progressive move by a Republican president known for supporting strict border enforcement to keep drugs out of the United States. Many legislators are calling for further reform of mandatory minimum sentences for minor or first-time drug offenses. The act provides people convicted and sentenced under mandatory minimum sentencing guidelines prior to 2010, including minor drug offenders, with the chance to have their sentences shortened.

For those who are already addicted, ensuring they have access to the treatment they need is crucial. Treatment can be expensive, and addicts may be discouraged by the cost to even try to obtain it. Those who think the government shouldn't have to foot the bill should consider the costs that add up from long-term drug addiction—emergency medical care for overdose or accidental injury, medical care for long-term health complications, legal fees, lost productivity, and so on. Consider, too, that addiction affects our family, friends, and neighbors. We are all in this together.

We should recognize that treatment for addiction is the same as for any other chronic disease. Once you're addicted, you're always addicted. We may break the chemical dependence, but the mental dependence remains, and treatment may last the patient's entire life. We need to make addiction treatment more available and more accessible—get the word out about treatment, and get the addict to the treatment center.

To prevent future opioid addiction, let us move beyond the "opioids are bad" message. Opioids still have their place in medicine, and those suffering from pain should still have access to them. But let's stop demanding complete pain relief when pain does occur, especially with opioids as the method of choice. We don't necessarily need high-powered pain medication with high addictive potential for every instance of pain. It's okay to feel some pain—pain is part of life.

How to Relieve the Pain

Extrapolated from the 2016 National Health Interview Survey (NHIS) data, the CDC estimates that 50 million Americans—just over 20 percent of the adult population—live with chronic pain, with about 20 million having pain that is severe enough that it frequently limits life or work activities.[8] Chronic pain has been linked to restrictions in mobility, lost productivity because of inability to work or perform daily activities, anxiety and depression, increased direct medical costs, and, as we have been discussing, dependence on opioids.

There is no one-size-fits-all approach to chronic pain, but the best is a multimodal one that includes physical therapy, changes in behavior, medication, and strategies that help people accept pain. Physicians tend to resort to drug therapy because it is easy, it's the only thing they have time to do, and, frankly, it is what the patient prefers. This is something we absolutely must change. We should also consider the question, is there a level of pain that is acceptable? Most people will have some form of age-related disease at some point, and some of that will come with discomfort. We have to be wary of masking all pain, as pain is the body's way of sending us a signal. We should also be wary of keeping pain so low that it requires continuous and often increasing doses of medications. Not only can this worsen a person's ability to function but it may also lead to medication misuse.

We have addicts in our country suffering and dying every day, and it's a huge problem. We won't solve the addiction problem by throwing each of them in jail or suing the physicians and pharmaceutical companies. True, the money gained may provide resources to help with addiction treatment, yet how much of it will actually trickle down to the person overdosing in an alleyway?

Lessening the monetary gain of enormous pharmaceutical companies will do little to prevent new cases of addiction. We need to help these people heal while at the same time implementing new restrictions on opioid access (legal and illegal). It all comes down to this bedrock American value: our nation allows everyone the opportunity to strive to better themselves. This includes people struggling with addiction. Let's lift them up and help them see that a better life is still possible through hard work and perseverance.

Chapter 7

THE AFFORDABLE
CARE ACT

A Self-Destructing System

We all have the right to life as our Declaration of Independence says. We also want to make sure all Americans have the opportunity to live their best lives. We can extrapolate from the right to life, liberty, and the pursuit of happiness that we also have a right to medical care, because to chase life, one must also pursue health. However, the right to medical care doesn't mean we have a right to *free medical care*. We also require food, water, and shelter to live, yet we don't demand that they be given to us gratis.

The Affordable Care Act is in part based on the idea that health insurance should cover all health care costs, including for illnesses or conditions we had prior to purchasing insurance. In fact, this is one of the ACA's most popular provisions: you cannot be denied coverage or be required to pay more because of a preexisting condition. However, this contradicts the basic function of insurance: to insure against the possibility of a *future* illness or condition. Under the ACA, health insurance is not really insurance at all—it's a reimbursement of medical costs incurred. However, I question whether all preexisting conditions should be lumped together.

The ACA also, in order to get more people covered by insurance, greatly expanded Medicaid, a program that was originally designed to provide coverage only for people at the bottom of the financial ladder. Medicaid expansion has entailed slashing physician compensation, onerous administrative costs, and propping up an overpriced drug industry through government subsidies. Not only has it put the American health care system on an unsustainable path financially, but it simultaneously banished the role of personal responsibility in the pursuit of a healthy life.

The Costs of the Affordable Care Act

The implementation of the Affordable Care Act in 2010 contributed to the drastic rise in employer costs by mandating which employers must offer health insurance benefits (based on factors like the number of employees) and what types of coverage those insurance plans must offer, termed "essential health benefits." Employers to which the mandates apply face penalties if they don't make coverage available that meets minimum value and affordability standards. As a result, to keep overall costs down, employers pushed more financial responsibility onto their employees in the form of high-deductible plans requiring increased out-of-pocket payments. Together, the provisions for employer mandates, expansion of Medicaid, and elimination of preexisting conditions restrictions led to higher costs for everyone. Employees' total financial responsibility (premiums, deductibles, and co-pays) increased by 54 percent from 2006 to 2016 while wages increased by only 29 percent during the same years, according to data from the Peterson-Kaiser Health System Tracker.[1] Although offset by a decrease in co-pays, the spending on deductibles alone rose 176 percent in the same time period with a notably sharp increase in 2010 at the time of ACA's passage.[2]

The ACA ended up replacing insurance with a weak attempt at socialized medicine. Its seismic impact on the private insurance market has continued to be felt a decade after its enactment, with insurance premiums for individual coverage more than doubling between 2013 and 2019. The average family premium is now over $19,000 a year, according to the National Conference of State Legislatures.[3] Out-of-pocket deductible spending has also grown sharply, with over 10 million people spending more than 10 percent of their income on premium costs and out-of-pocket expenses, according to the Commonwealth Fund.[4]

Yes, the ACA may have slightly slowed health care spending since its inception, but was the slowdown because of increased out-of-pocket costs for average Americans? To continue the trend of allowing a cash drain, in 2020, the Internal Revenue Service set out-of-pocket limits for family coverage at $16,300, which is up from 2019 ($15,800) and significantly above that in 2014 ($12,700).[5] The continued increase of out-of-pocket maximums is a system to keep premiums in check to feed the talking point of "premiums are stabilizing"; however, according to a 2018 analysis by Wyman Actuarial Consulting, insurance premiums will continue to rise another 2 percent in 2020 "if the IRS implements the [ACA] tax as planned."[6] The ACA health insurance industry fee, intended to fund the ACA's marketplace exchanges, has been delayed out of fear that there may be further premium increases; without it, the long-term stability of the ACA is in jeopardy. However, the fee undermines the fundamental ideology of limited government. It is essentially an annual tax on health insurance companies based on their market share, something that again calls to mind the bodega owner paying protection money to the mafia to hold property on a block.

In addition to the implementation of this tax, a change in premium tax credits is eventual and may further raise premiums for more than 7 million Americans, according to CBPP estimates.[7] Basically, insurance is set to become a lot more expensive for those not receiving subsidies under the ACA, much like middle-class America. Also, those needing to purchase individual plans on the ACA exchanges will continue to have limited choices. The ability to choose has not been a dominant theme in the chronicle of the Affordable Care Act marketplace. In fact, there were several potential "bare counties" that had only a single option for coverage, according to early predictions.[8] Some insurers looked at their balance sheets and pulled out altogether; an analysis done by Kaiser showed that, in 2019, some states had only one insurer, which isn't really a choice at all.[9] The combination of "over-entry" from the expansion, "under-paying" from tax credits, and cost-sharing reductions continue to contribute to the instability.

When there is limited choice in a private market, there is no price competition, which causes prices to increase. The Trump administration claimed its primary goal for health care is improved access and increased choice. Holding true to this claim, it has lessened the restrictions of the ACA to enable private health insurers to offer more affordable plans based on varying coverage options. In doing so, this has contributed to a recent increase in insurers offering options on the exchange, including a few less expensive plans.[10]

However, the bottom line remains, if you do not qualify for federal subsidies to offset the overall increased cost of health insurance, the Affordable Care Act is not actually affordable. The increased prices across the country for comprehensive health care plans are really cost sharing to subsidize those who have preexisting conditions or no health insurance at all. To meet the ACA requirements for all-inclusive policies, insurance companies have had to charge more to help cover the cost for patients with expensive chronic diseases. For those who make too much money to qualify for Medicaid but not enough to buy their own plans, the government—that is, the taxpayer—has to step in to subsidize the costs.

This isn't single-payer health care—*yet*. As health insurance continues to be exorbitantly expensive, and Americans continue on a path of poor dietary and lifestyle habits leading to chronic diseases, the government will further subsidize through more taxes to pay for increasing disease prevalence.

While it's true that the Affordable Care Act (ACA) extended health insurance to millions of Americans, this was largely through subsidies and the expansion of Medicaid. In other words, the ACA is a bailout without reparation of the underlying issues.

Overuse of the ED

Supporters of the law claimed people who have health insurance are more likely to seek preventative care from their primary-care physician and rely less on costly emergency departments (ED); therefore, also more likely to have diseases caught early, when treatment is less costly. So why didn't the increase in insurance coverage cause a decrease in expensive emergency room visits? While nearly 20 million Americans gained insurance coverage, the number of primary-care physicians to treat them did not increase. In particular, people with Medicaid had difficulty finding physicians who would accept it—many won't provide care for the nominal reimbursements typically offered by Medicaid. Therefore, just as before, emergency departments fill the gap. They remain overcrowded because they treat all patients, whether they have private insurance, government insurance, or no insurance at all. This has now led to the large insurance companies dictating not only which hospitals you can visit as a fully covered patient but also which conditions are allowable to be treated by emergency physicians.

Here's the problem: patients aren't very good at judging if a symptom is an emergency or not. Let's take the person with a severe headache who goes to the ED only to learn he has a migraine that will go away with a little rest and relaxation and an over-the-counter pain reliever. Still, that person was seen by a number of ED personnel: the visit costs money. To counteract the high costs of emergency care for nonemergent conditions, some insurance companies are now saying that if your condition turns out to be nonemergent, like a migraine, then your ED visit won't be covered by insurance and you'll have to foot the hefty bill yourself.

This sounds reasonable to the extent that we want to decrease non-urgent cases in the emergency departments. Take another person who has a severe headache who does not seek medical treatment. However, this person never wakes up because the headache was in fact caused by a ruptured brain aneurysm. Migraines and ruptured brain aneurysms both present with severe headaches. If insurance companies continue telling the insured that their care won't be covered if it's not an "emergency," and those people steer clear of the ED as a result, then they may be taking dangerous risks with their health. This rationing of covered care and gambling with life have surpassed the boundaries of health insurance.

The Failure of the Individual Mandate

The ACA requires insurers to cover everyone and charge them the same rates, without price adjusting for their anticipated cost of treatment. That's well-intentioned but what does it do? It encourages people to wait until they need coverage to sign up. This leaves the insurance pool disproportionately composed of sick patients—and thus yields higher premiums for everyone.

In an effort to reduce this phenomena, a coverage mandate was developed. Many Americans rejected the notion of the individual mandate, which required that all Americans have health insurance or pay a financial penalty. Because of this, the tax reform package passed by the Republican Congress and signed by President Trump in 2017 struck down the mandate, a move applauded by conservatives, who viewed the mandate as unconstitutional. Eliminating the mandate led to the first decrease in the number of insured since implementation of the ACA. That's right: individuals—many of them young and healthy—are choosing to gamble and not have health insurance now that there is no financial penalty. Why shouldn't they take that gamble? Under the existing rules of the ACA, they can put off buying an insurance plan until they actually need medical care.

Here is the problem: this leads to a paucity of young, healthy people in the insurance pool to balance out older or sicker people more likely to need costly medical care. Unfortunately, when cost sharing is high, meaning high-deductible plans, the people with these plans are nearly as likely as the uninsured to skip needed care, such as filling prescriptions or going to the doctor when they are sick. So, the numbers may show that people have gained coverage, but with rising deductibles and premiums, they are less likely to use it.

This is the ACA flaw that must be rectified immediately to avoid catastrophe. President Obama and the ACA's supporters didn't understand the need to incentivize people, especially the young and healthy, to maintain continuous health insurance coverage. Instead they approached it from the wrong end, threatening penalties for not having insurance. People who maintain insurance should not be penalized with a rise in premiums or restricted coverage when they do eventually require medical care as they are now. However, for people who choose not to maintain insurance but then purchase it at the last minute because they need services, their premiums should reflect the higher cost of insuring them. Reward the people who demonstrate responsibility, and discipline those who don't. It really is that simple. The ACA blanket penalty for the uninsured only made costs go up for everyone.

Socialization of Health Care

The ACA was a flawed start to impose semi-socialized government health insurance on America. It disrupted the health insurance industry and did little to rein in the costs of the system itself.

The Trump administration, working with Congress, has taken some steps to mitigate these problems, but it will take congressional action to yield long-term, effective results. The lack of bipartisan consensus in Congress will undoubtedly put America on the path toward a single-payer system out of default and frustration. The cry for universal health care by progressive Democrats is only getting louder as presidential candidates make empty, pie-in-the-sky campaign promises of Medicare-for-All. All of this is ironic considering that Democrats were hell-bent on saving the ACA up to now. Former vice president Joe Biden, the most pragmatic Democrat at this point, is one of the only party leaders continuing to push to improve the ACA rather than throw it out in favor of single-payer. The truth is, single-payer is not very popular. Americans understand that a massive tax increase would be required to pay for it, not to mention the fact that many are satisfied with their employer-provided insurance and don't want to be forced to give it up. They also know that tens of trillions of tax dollars dedicated to government health care would mean the government has less revenue to spend on other segments of our economy.

Beyond the double-digit increases in tax rates, implementing socialized medicine would exact a far greater human cost. A complete overhaul of the American health care system. The elimination of private insurance would result in further rationed care and hinder advances in treatment. Overall, Americans would have less money in their paychecks and will not be any healthier to show for it. A single, government-run system for a vast country of fifty individual states, each with its own diverse population, is not only unfeasible, it is inviting disaster.

As President Trump has himself admitted, health care is extremely complicated. A simple fact can guide us: Americans want to know that when they get sick, they will have access to high-quality medical care, and that they won't go broke paying for it.

Policy masterminds continue to throw around various versions of the same concept to provide affordable, accessible health care for all Americans. However, whether we reform or replace Obamacare, the fundamental issue of overutilization remains. The ACA functions to increase coverage but it involves lowering access to care for many, increased costs, and lessening physician reimbursement. This may result in more insurance coverage, but does it leave us with a system Americans even want?

Dismantling the ACA

In the first two years of President Trump's presidency, the Republican-led Congress made multiple failed attempts to repeal the ACA and come up with a viable new health care policy. The only success on that front was the GOP tax reform bill, which undid the individual mandate. This led to the question of whether the rest of the ACA would fall apart without it. As for now, it appears that the ACA is here to stay.

Reinsurance Programs

The biggest complaint under the ACA has been that it was supposed to bring down premiums and out-of-pocket costs but failed to do so for many Americans. In 2019, Maryland was able to decrease insurance premiums across all health insurance plans by means of a reinsurance program. On the surface this seems to suggest that the ACA had finally stabilized, but in fact this apparent success came with increased deductibles. Federal reinsurance programs have been tried before with the same results, according to the Cato Institute.[11] It is a case of robbing Peter to pay Paul: the data show lower premiums, yes, but also higher deductibles and/or co-pays along with higher taxes to maintain state government funding.

If Maryland experiences something similar to what happened at the national level, insurance companies in Maryland will quickly note that the state is offering substantially lower subsidies than requested to cover costs. In other words, the reinsurance program is a government bailout for insurance companies required by the ACA to offer high-cost comprehensive plans. The insurance companies raise out-of-pocket payments for consumers to cover the cost of preexisting conditions. This is a recipe for disaster that will only burden people with the same problems presented by the ACA—drastically increased premiums and deductibles when the government doesn't pay up. If it does, there will be a huge political fallout as taxpayers are again asked to foot the bill for failed policies.

The very idea that federal subsidies of any kind reduce the cost of premiums is the exact fabrication Washington will forever proclaim. It serves not only the economic interests of insurance companies but also the political interests of politicians who want to come across as "taking action" when in fact they are not fixing anything. Rather than focus on government bailouts for the ACA, the Trump administration has taken action at the individual level.

Puzzle Pieces

In order to indemnify the individual financial burden, some restrictions on tax-free contributions to Health Savings Accounts (HSAs) have been lifted by the Trump administration. This is a smart move. However, HSA funds still cannot be used for insurance premiums, making it essential either to lower premiums or further expand HSAs. HSAs put the responsibility on the consumer to make decisions about their medical care; they encourage price-shopping and limiting nonessential visits to the doctor while reducing premiums. On the other hand, account holders are restricted to insurers' limited networks, so price-shopping and "choice" occur more in theory than in practice.

In addition to expanding HSA use, another focus of Republican proposals include short-term catastrophic plans. Catastrophic plans insure against the costs of serious illness or injuries but not ordinary, everyday health issues. Because these insurance plans are less comprehensive than those required under the ACA, they are more affordable. Most often these plans are sought by younger (healthier) adults and those aging out of their parents' plans who do not have employer-based coverage and cannot yet afford the larger programs required by the ACA.

The insurance company lobbyists argue catastrophic plans siphon off healthier patients from the larger pool, therefore ultimately driving up premiums for others. They are right. Here is where the fundamental question arises: Should younger and healthier people trying to get their feet on the ground shoulder the cost burden of older, sicker people? Doesn't it behoove us to support the younger generation and give them ample opportunity to be successful? The alternative is that they won't purchase any health insurance because they can't afford it, which would still keep them out of the larger health insurance pool.

Ultimately, Americans want choice. A proposal often voiced by those on the right is to allow people to buy insurance plans across state lines, which would increase competition among insurance companies in different regions and, ideally, provide more affordable options for everyone. Will this solve the bigger problem of continued rising costs? No. But it is another small piece to a very large and complex puzzle.

The Impact of Medicaid Expansion

Nearly 14 million adults gained Medicaid coverage under the Affordable Care Act. Efforts to repeal the ACA failed largely because of the popularity of this expansion. In states that participated in Medicaid expansion (not all did), the program now covers people with incomes below 138 percent of the federal poverty level.

This is a departure from traditional Medicaid, which provided health insurance coverage for low-income Americans (up to 133 FPL). Over the years since its inception in 1965, it was expanded to cover care for the disabled, nursing home care for the aged, and other categories. Most people are under the impression Medicare will pay for a nursing home, but in fact Medicare covers only a maximum of three days after a hospital admission, then Medicaid kicks in. With increased life expectancy, 50 to 70 percent of people can expect to require significant long-term care when they pass age sixty-five. According to the Congressional Budget Office, long-term care expenditures in 2000 totaled $30 billion; by 2015 that number had climbed to $225 billion, half of which is paid for by Medicaid. Unfortunately, government intrusion into health care has made the nursing home issue more fraught. Patients are discharged faster from the hospital to control costs, which means that potentially sicker patients go into skilled-nursing facilities requiring care that should have been provided in the hospital. Additionally, with funding allocated to the millions of additional people covered under the Medicaid expansion, there is less available for others. Yes, more people are covered, but the disbursement amount is rationed.

Until now the federal share of the Medicaid expansion under the ACA was 100 percent, and as such, according to North Carolina governor Roy Cooper's budget proposal for 2019–2020, Medicaid expansion will deplete federal funds by $1.91 billion. In 2020 the federal share will drop to 90 percent, and barring a change to the law, it will stay there. This creates a balancing act for state budgets: states will have to determine whether the Medicaid expansion actually reduces spending on uncompensated medical services or, now that they are responsible for 10 percent of the expansion, will they have to raise state taxes, too?

One can argue that, overall, Medicaid expansion brought positive change because millions more Americans obtained health insurance, but it had negative impacts outside of the obvious tax burden. For one thing, health care providers faced a rapid increase in the volume of people seeking care. People newly eligible for Medicaid lost the incentive to obtain insurance on their own as they got used to receiving government assistance. In California, where nearly one in three residents are on Medicaid, the growth of this entitlement, like most other entitlements, has proven unsustainable. Rather than making yet more people dependent on government, shouldn't we be trying to move people into the private sector and promote financial independence? Undoubtedly, our health system has many holes, and the Medicaid program helps plug those holes. However, far too many Americans are reliant on this subsidy, which dilutes funding for those for whom Medicaid was originally developed. Any hope to reform Medicaid and restore fiscal sustainability to the program will require reducing waste and abuse of the system as well as supporting its recipients and helping them to succeed without government assistance.

A more conservative approach to making a sustainable Medicaid is seeking to ensure that the system is fiscally responsible. Seema Verma, a health policy expert appointed by President Trump to head the Centers for Medicare and Medicaid Services, worked on the redesign of Indiana's Medicaid program before going to Washington. Her innovations included cost sharing with funded HSA accounts for Medicaid consumers. Traditionally, Medicaid patients paid no premiums and either nominal or no co-pays; this ultimately led to a failing program because of overuse of health services, the lack of both positive and negative reinforcements for maintaining wellness, and fraud.

As CMS administrator, Verma pressed work requirements for able-bodied adults receiving Medicaid benefits. Though this was a controversial stance, she was well aware that the trajectory of Medicaid is unsustainable without major reforms to rein in spending. Either eligibility needs to be limited, or those who are eligible need to be encouraged to make some kind of contribution to society rather than simply receive entitlements. Work requirements would do just that. Although employed Medicaid recipients might still be unable to afford comprehensive private health insurance, they would demonstrate responsibility through work, thus contributing to our overall workforce and paying taxes.

The concept of work requirements remains tied up in legal (and moral) debate. One side claims that most people want to work but are unable to find a job, and that they should not be barred from insurance coverage because of that. The other side claims that the economy is booming, with more job openings than job seekers. However, those in need of a job may not have the requisite skills and training. To remedy the skills gap, the government could operate a data base of entry-level jobs and other positions of varying skill levels. This would benefit both the unemployed and employers and would cost taxpayers a lot less than doling out more subsidies.

Lastly, the current funding method for Medicaid is a fee-for-service system, in which the federal government meets the states' requests. States are subjected to only limited oversight; they alone determine who is eligible for coverage, and the federal government has historically complied. If the states were required to take a closer look at their own Medicaid programs with an eye toward reducing costs, it would benefit the states' other publicly funded programs and also reduce the national debt burden. The introduction of state block grants would force each state to make their budgets work with a fixed sum of federal money. This would encourage states, which are most familiar with their own populations, to offer coverage to those who need it most. With block grants rather than fee-for-service, the states would not only find ways to eliminate excess spending and reduce Medicaid waste, but they would place national health spending on a more sustainable path.

According to the CMS, in 2016 waste, abuse, and fraud in the Medicaid system accounted for nearly $140 billion, or 12 percent of Medicaid spending, a rate that doubled in only a few short years following the ACA's liberalization of Medicaid eligibility rules.[12] To compensate for this waste, federal and state legislators have clamored to reduce health care compensation for services by increasing the use of nurses and technicians rather than physicians for medical services. Ultimately, these moves are lowering the quality of medical care for Americans everywhere.

Slashing Physician Compensation

While it is true that physicians in the United States are paid more than those in any other country, reducing the amount we pay them for their services will only leave us chasing our tails. If we continue to replace our highly trained physicians with midlevel caregivers with a fraction of the training, the resultant cost savings will be nominal. Physician compensation is mistakenly regarded as accounting for the bulk of medical costs when in fact their salaries account for only 8 percent of overall health care expenditure in the United States.[13] Even if doctors worked for free this would not make a dent in lowering the cost of health care in this country given the fact that in 2018 the government spent over $1 trillion on health care alone.[14]

Yet, in order to pay for the increased use of our system, specialty physicians' reimbursements are decreasing. This is not a good thing. Doctors spend an average of 40,000 hours in training (undergraduate degree, medical degree, residency/fellowship of 3–9 years depending on specialty at approximately 80 hours per week): that's roughly equivalent to twenty years of full-time work before they even start earning in their profession.[15] In addition, in 2018 the average medical student graduated with $196,520 in debt with three to nine years of training still to go before receiving attending-level compensation.[16] Do we really want to be punitive to those who dedicate the most time to being experts in their field? Each reimbursement decrease moves us away from the "hard work pays off" culture. Rather than punishing our doctors, let's focus on the real factors raising our costs.

High Administrative Costs

In addition to the criticism of insurance companies and physician salaries, supporters of single-payer point to the high administrative costs of the American system. Our complex payment scheme involving multiple payers, public and private, as well as varying reimbursement rates causes systemic fragmentation. All of which leads to high administrative costs, accounting for 25 percent of hospital spending.[17] The billing and electronic health record (EHR) requirements under the ACA made matters worse.

A higher level of complexity means more time and effort are required to process claims. However, a distinguishing feature of the American health system is that it offers a plethora of choice, including which doctor you see and when, as well as which health insurance plan you purchase. At least, that was true before the ACA. Additionally, as patients are required to pay more money out-of-pocket under the ACA, medical practices and hospitals have needed more resources to collect unpaid bills, which further adds to the costs.

Single-payer is thus touted as the gold standard for eliminating these administrative charges. However, billing complexity varies dramatically among insurers across the country, with Medicaid being more complex and difficult to bill than any other insurers. Complexity of billing, including the time to payment, number of interactions between physician and payer, and intricate coding input, leads to improper denial of claims, which mires all parties in further negotiations and paperwork. In fact, Medicaid's claim denial rate is much higher than that of Medicare and private insurers.[18] Yet this convoluted, restrictive system would be 100 percent of claims if single-payer was implemented in the United States.

Rather than a complete government takeover, the ACA called for unification and automation of an electronic health system to reduce administrative costs. Health information technology (HIT) and EHR were intended to streamline administrative tasks and patient care, resulting in long-term cost savings. However, the use of HIT and EHR not only imposed a cost burden on the system but led to less doctor/patient interaction and longer off-hour computer work for doctors. Matters only got more complicated but not cheaper.[19]

Reducing health care administrative costs in the United States would have direct and indirect impacts on the entire system. The most obvious impact would be the direct monetary savings resulting from cutting back wasteful spending from unnecessary activities. Each year, health care payers and providers in the United States spend about $496 billion on billing and insurance-related costs, according to the Center for American Progress. If that number isn't shocking enough, a 2010 report by the National Academy of Medicine estimated that half of that is waste.[20]

Still, even if we were to adopt a single-payer system like Canada's, according to a thorough study by the National Academy of Medicine, we would decrease the cost of health care by, at most, 14.4 percent, only to be counterbalanced by a hefty rise in taxes.[21] Although 14 percent of the $3.6 trillion we spend on administrative tasks equates to a lot of money ($504 billion), it is not enough to foot the single-payer bill and would leave us with a system that would not benefit the American consumer. Rather, identifying the causes of administrative waste, implementing change to counter it, and focusing on other means to lower the overall cost of health care seems far more practical than a complete overhaul of our system.[22]

The High Cost of Drugs

Americans spend more on prescription drugs than our global counterparts, averaging roughly $1,200 per person per year.[23] Although the high prices of pharmaceuticals in the United States are controversial, pharmaceutical companies say that high revenues are critical to innovation, including the development of potentially lifesaving drugs. Americans do pay more for their medications, but it's also true that the United States leads the world in cancer survival in part because it is a top innovator in development of cancer drug treatments, to which Americans have wide access. Very expensive cancer treatments such as the new immunotherapies are more available in America than in countries with nationalized systems that set restrictions on drug access based on cost-benefit analyses and budget caps.[24]

Nevertheless, the high cost of prescription drugs is a serious problem, and the ACA did the minimum to fix it. "Financial toxicity" is a term that refers to problems patients face in paying for medical care and is often used in relation to cancer patients for whom the costs of care can be particularly high. The financial burdens imposed on those suffering from cancer and other ailments raise serious questions about who we are as a country. If drug prices continue their current trajectory, then we will be on the path to making decisions about who will live and who will die. Drastic measures will need to be taken because we won't have the resources to treat everyone. If we adopt universal health care, then these innovative therapies will only be readily available to those who can afford to pay for them, so that is not the answer.

When a doctor prescribes an expensive medication for an insured patient, the insurance company responds in one of three ways:

1. The insurance company pays for the medication, which ultimately adds to the rising costs of insurance premiums.
2. The insurance company pays for a portion of the medication and the patient pays for the rest as an out-of-pocket expense. If the patient has a robust HSA, this may cover it, but it may also drain the account.
3. The insurance company denies the claim and the patient is responsible for the entire cost.

When the second and third scenarios occur, often patients will not get the prescription filled, and consequently not take the medication as prescribed. Even more often, the prescribing doctor is unaware that the patient must cover a large share of the cost of the medication, and assumes the patient is taking it when they are not.

Frequently, there are more affordable medications that will work the same for the medical condition being treated. However, the prices differ depending on the insurance company's relationship with a pharmacy benefit manager (PBM) and the rebates that were negotiated. PBMs, the middlemen between the pharmaceutical companies and the insurance companies, are one of the least regulated and least understood facets of our pharmaceutical delivery network. They also grew to become a dominant force under the ACA. Initially, PBMs offered lower drug prices by negotiating with pharmaceutical companies and creating alliances with insurance companies. However, now that many of these under-the-radar PBMs have coalesced to form larger entities, prices have risen. PBMs arbitrarily increase prices and then provide a rebate, but this is merely a bait-and-switch tactic that complicates the system and disrupts patient care by requiring prior authorizations and restricting the medications that will be covered.

In this ploy, the normal feedback loops of a free market don't exist. Minimizing the role of PBMs in our medication delivery system will not only lower costs and administrative waste but reduce the delay in care that so many experience because of worries about cost. Reducing waste is key, not hindering advancement.

It's inarguably true that drug prices are too high in the United States, but we should not be so quick to make negative comparisons to Europe. First, over 57 percent of pharmaceutical R&D happens in the United States. In Europe, government-driven monopolies on drug prices lead to price fixing, which naturally drives down profitability for the pharmaceutical companies. The same companies raise drug prices in the United States to counteract the loss. In considering how to bring down drug prices, we have to be careful not to inhibit expensive but vital innovation.

Investments in science are critical to support a robust drug pipeline. For biopharmaceuticals, patents are a driver for development, ensuring companies are investing in lifesaving medicines. In March 2019, New Jersey senator Cory Booker said in a CNN Democratic presidential town hall event that "we're going to take away your patent and let the generics come in and undercut those prices." But we must be careful when dealing with intellectual property rights. These companies must justify their investments, so protecting their patents is essential.

Promoting healthy competition in the generics and biosimilars markets, however, is a chief component that needs to be carefully looked at. On one hand, limiting competition can lead to spiked prices and drug shortages, but on the other hand, not safeguarding patents can reduce development. The best policy will be somewhere in the middle.

One government solution is to shorten patents' duration and put regulations on the market share companies are able to acquire. Historically, leading drug companies will often extend their patents and block others from entering the market. Or when their patent is expiring, they will spike prices as a last push for profit. Price controls in the manner of socialist systems are no solution. Instead we should think outside the box to find a different incentive structure that not only encourages future R&D by protecting intellectual property but expands on patent protections. An idea could be creating a licensing strategy that would allow drug companies to capture profit from the generic market as well if they are engaged in additional R&D. Positive incentives will bring less costly generics to the market while protecting American capitalism. A functioning generics market is vital to providing patients with affordable access to needed drugs. However, when we talk about access to treatments and services, the focus is consistently on increasing supply, potentially at the expense of R&D, whereas the same effect could be had if we decreased the demand by reducing illness.

Supply vs. Demand

Health services spending can be broken down principally as a function of prices and utilization. Economists focus their criticism on rising health care prices, but what if the rising prices are closer to being on par with our evolving medical technologies? For most of the 1980s and 1990s, health care price growth in the United States outpaced utilization of health care services. Price growth then slowed in the 2000s with the recession, and after the Affordable Care Act, utilization became the dominant driver of spending because of the millions of people added to the ranks of the insured (the majority through the Medicaid expansion).

As we have discussed, the CDC tells us that 80 percent of all deaths from heart disease are attributable to preventable factors such as being overweight, not enough exercise, alcohol intake, and poor diet. When it comes to health insurance costs, do we put all disease in the same basket? Do we separate out the obese patient who needs gastric bypass surgery or expensive cholesterol-lowering medications from the young mother diagnosed with breast cancer and found to have a genetic mutation predisposing her to that cancer? Or the lifelong heavy smoker diagnosed with advanced lung cancer from the ten-year-old diagnosed with insulin-dependent type 1 diabetes? The ACA's preexisting condition policy does not distinguish between preventable and unavoidable disease. Doesn't it make sense to reduce demand for health care services for preventable disease, rather than only focusing on cheapening the supply? Could that become the focus of budget critics?

Access to care is not the same thing as comprehensive health insurance and coverage of preexisting conditions. Health insurance is for a disease that has not yet formed. Of course patients with preexisting conditions should have access to care; one way to ensure this may be with the use of high-risk pools and block grants to states.

Risk pooling is grouping together individuals at all levels of risk, whose medical costs are combined to calculate premiums. This action allows the higher costs of the less healthy to be offset by the lower costs of the healthy. The ACA applied this concept of leveling the playing field to all levels of risk through the preexisting conditions requirements and cost of coverage restrictions, which is why premiums rose for the majority of Americans. According to the Kaiser Family Foundation, the sickest group of Americans are only 5 percent of the population and account for over 50 percent of all health care expenditures.[25] That means the rest of us are compensating for their cost through higher premiums and cost sharing. An alternative approach would be to direct external funding, in the form of block grants, to high-risk pools, a grouping of people all at higher risk for health problems. This would guarantee funding for the most infirm and could also lower the costs for the healthy. Block grants are fixed amounts that the federal government allocates to states for a specific purpose. If Medicaid was turned into a block grant, the federal government would set each state's Medicaid spending amount in advance. This would force the states to control their Medicaid budgets, as previously discussed.

Let us remember that traditional insurance proved successful by charging risk-based premiums with causality negating payout. When did health insurance morph from this paradigm of protection for potential illness to complete coverage for all medical conditions—comprehensive coverage without financial culpability, regardless of the cause of illness? Politicians, economists, and pundits may blame the rise in health care costs on drug makers, doctors, and hospital administration, but what if we are causing the rising costs?

The Big Picture Ignored by the ACA

According to a 2016 study, less than 3 percent of Americans are living a healthy lifestyle (getting enough exercise, eating a good diet, not having too much body fat, and not smoking).[26]

Our poor health may be bankrupting our nation. The majority of our medical cost is from chronic diseases, and half of them are preventable.

It is time to face it: we are the problem with our health care system.

We are an industrious people who work hard at our jobs.

We value education, and we work hard at that, too.

But we don't work hard to maintain our health. We don't take steps—even easy ones—to prevent disease.

To improve our health care economy, we need to focus on our individual choices. If we can't control the growth of health care spending by controlling ourselves, the problems will extend beyond the health sector. If health care spending sends us over a fiscal cliff, we'll wish we spent more time worrying about individual and national accountability in finance and health.

Cardiovascular disease and stroke account for nearly 20 percent of all health expenditures. In 2018, health expenditures on these diseases, combined with lost productivity, totaled more than $329 billion.[27] It is consistently demonstrated that about 80 percent of deaths from heart disease and stroke can be attributed to preventable factors such as obesity, low physical activity, heavy drinking, and poor diet.[28]

	$3.3 T total cost	Cost attributed to preventable disease	Cost of unavoidable illness
CV Disease/ Stroke	$329B	$263B	$66B
Cancer	$147B	$62B	$85B

Estimated national expenditures for cancer care in the United States in 2017 were $147.3 billion. In future years, costs are likely to increase as the population ages and cancer prevalence increases. Costs are also likely to increase as new, and often more expensive, treatments are adopted as standards of care.[29]

Rising health care prices are not a new phenomenon. They do not represent an unavoidable cataclysm about which we can do nothing other than hide our heads. To solve our crisis, we don't need to look to oppressive, statist policies, but to ourselves. We must use our freedoms and individual choices to bring about solutions.

When will we realize that we don't have to adopt socialism to stave off the cost of our bad behaviors, but rather resolve to be a healthier society? We can still continue to lead the world in innovation in health care if we would only commit to lowering our own cost of care. Together, as a society, we need to make hard choices to reach such goals and stop expecting the government and our doctors to fix the mess we have made. The ACA handed out insurance like candy and wrongfully placed the burden of diminishing disease on the medical doctors rather than on the individual. Now we are all becoming increasingly aware of the consequences.

Chapter 8

THE MEDICAL
DOCTOR

A Dying Profession

As an institution, the medical profession is in crisis. Doctors no longer command the respect they once did. The increasing demands of an overburdened system have made their difficult jobs even more so. Doctors are people, too, and few realize just how intense the stress of the profession has become.

Until recently, people grew up going to their family physician's office. You knew everyone well, from the receptionist to the doctor. Now, we have pop-up urgent care centers in our street-corner pharmacies, where there's a new person every day to provide medical evaluations—and it's often not even a doctor.

The depersonalization of medicine has followed the changes in other aspects of daily life—gone are the days where "everybody knows your name" at the local bar or coffee shop, or we have a long-standing relationship with the barber who cuts our hair or the mechanic who works on our car. Unfortunately, fostering personal relationships and developing trust do not seem to be the future of America.

Loss of Respect

Once upon a time, patients followed doctors' orders. You'd go to a doctor with a complaint, the doctor would tell you what to do, and you'd do it. Not anymore. The very notion of a doctor telling the patient what to do is perceived as paternalistic, or even condescending.

In college, I studied microbiology and Spanish. When you live in Arizona, knowing Spanish is very important, so that's what made me pursue it in school. It eventually became an asset, because I could speak to patients without having to call interpreters.

One night during my first year of residency, an older Hispanic woman came into the hospital with a form of chronic disease that wasn't being managed well at home. She spoke only Spanish.

It was the middle of the night, and she and her family came in together. As I was speaking to her in Spanish, with her whole family present, she refused to respond to me. Her reaction toward me was almost hostile, to the point where I was questioning my ability to communicate effectively with her. Could she understand what I was saying?

Her daughter pulled me aside and said, "She feels you are disrespecting her by speaking such a formal version of her language." I was dumbfounded. I thought that eliminating the third-party interpreter and speaking Spanish to the patient myself not only would be appreciated but also viewed as friendly rather than standoffish. I explained to her daughter that I learned formal Castilian Spanish in college and was never in an immersion program. The Spanish I knew was useful for studying Spanish poetry and architecture, but apparently not for conversation.

She told me, "I think that's the problem." She said her mother spoke an informal Mexican dialect, so it seemed condescending for me to speak to her in formal Spanish.

It took me a minute to understand what she was saying. It was as though I were speaking the Queen's English to someone in South Carolina. They're both English, but they're extremely different dialects.

Regardless of the reason, I no longer speak Spanish to my patients. I wait for an available translator in an effort not to offend anymore. It may not be the best way to communicate with patients, but we are in a diverse nation and it's the best we can do. As a physician, you want to have a relationship with your patients without causing offense. What struck me about my perfect Spanish grammar being taken as offensive was that, at one point, it was okay for a physician to have a paternalistic tone.

The Rushed Office Visit

What we are seeing now is that people want to be an active member of their health care team. I'm a huge advocate for that. However, even embracing the teamwork concept isn't working. Our problem is the chronic lack of time and effort on the part of physicians and patients alike.

The average length of a visit with a primary-care doctor ranges from eight to eighteen minutes. That's saying "hello," getting out your most pressing concerns, and talking about the plan. To be efficient, the doctor must control the conversation. There's going to be no back and forth, and there's less time for listening and discussing topics, such as medication reviews and potential preventative care, let alone assessing someone's mental health.

You go to see your doctor because your knee hurts, and she gives you a brace and medication for it. You don't talk about why your knee is hurting or what you've been doing for it. You may not even discuss the benefits of physical therapy or if there is something you can do to prevent the pain from occurring. You probably won't ask about the risks and benefits of the medication to make sure you're okay with the potential side effects and costs. And when's the last time you and your doctor had the time to talk about what you're eating, your exercise regimen, and your work life to see if any of it is a contributing factor to your knee pain?

The less time we spend in the doctor's office, the less we're having those conversations. We're practicing reactive medicine. We talk about fixing (or just temporarily relieving) the pain and then we're finished. Even if we did have more time available, that's not necessarily what every patient wants anymore. Patients, like everyone else, want to be in and out and don't really want their doctors telling them what to do. Sadly, physicians lack modern-day units to combat the demise of a previously revered profession.

The American Medical Association: A Story of Treason

Since its founding in 1847, the American Medical Association has served as the self-appointed chief lobbying group *for* physicians, and it was initially made up of physicians. In 1910 the AMA started limiting the number of doctors that could be trained. It closed several medical schools that it declared were turning out substandard physicians—that's how it controlled the number of physicians to avoid diluting the market. Until the 1980s, no new medical schools could open.

Before the 1980s, the AMA made most of its revenue from physician dues. It cared about private physicians and, by extension, the practice of medicine and patient care in general.

Today, the AMA has changed entirely. Only 15 to 20 percent of practicing physicians are actual members of the AMA (I am not one of them). This is a huge decrease in membership over the last half century—in the 1950s, nearly 75 percent of doctors were members. Yet, despite the decreased involvement, the organization is doing better financially than it ever has. In the late 1980s, the AMA found that it was consistently losing money, never reporting more than $7.6 million in profit.[1] Yet starting with the turn of the new millennium, the AMA once again found itself profitable; in 2010, it reported an astounding $72 million in revenues from royalties of its products, twice as much as it took in for membership dues that year.[2]

So, what brilliant move in the 1980s led to the AMA's taking in more from the government than its own members? With government approval and funding, the AMA created a coding system, called the CPT codebook, that all doctors and hospitals were required to use to bill government and private insurance. As the codification of medicine required more and more paperwork, the AMA was more than happy to step in and supply the pricey systems to help the government and doctors—at a price, of course. All the while medical practices were mandated to purchase these expensive systems.

While the need for a centralized billing structure was obvious, the CPT system put forth by the AMA was not only self-servicing but redundant and complex. The billing codification abolished transparency in medical billing by swapping out procedures and diagnoses with numeric codes, which are required under the ACA billing rules. Had these codes been solidified, this may have worked. However, the coding changes require doctors, hospitals, and other health care systems to continuously update them annually. No wonder, with its vast lobbying power, the AMA supported the Affordable Care Act. The financial benefits were monumental and a sure way to bring in profits while membership continued to dwindle. Even after Democrats defaulted on the assurance of not allowing Medicare rates to further decrease.

Worse yet, the AMA became a strong arm of the government under what was called the Balanced Budget Act. In it, there was a fixed pot of money for physician reimbursement under government-funded health care. In theory, under the AMA—all specialty areas of medicine, like radiology and surgery and internal medicine—have representation. However, in the AMA's rules, if a specialty society doesn't maintain a certain level of AMA membership, it loses its seat on the bargaining committee. Therefore, if you're not paying your dues, you don't get a say in how much your specialty gets in medical reimbursements.

So, the AMA claims its top priority is helping doctors, but is it really?

The AMA may have grown too big for its own britches. Physicians are being squeezed out by an organization that was originally developed to maintain the doctor-patient relationship and preserve the quality of medicine. My, how times and profit-mongering have changed the association. The combination of the Affordable Care Act with its electronic health record requirements and the AMA with its CPT codes is causing small medical practices everywhere to close and forcing consolidation of the ones that remain open.

The Evolution of Physician Burnout

Doctors are told to be balanced, but spend a lifetime training not to be balanced and to ignore all signs of emotional, physical, and mental weakness in spite of the constantly changing professional landscape. To doctors, another word for fatigue is weakness. Ignore the exhaustion, and we aren't weak. For me, whatever symptom I am feeling, I tell myself I would rather have that than any of the cancer diagnoses I delivered that day, so I tell myself to buck up and move forward.

We don't focus on the thousands of cancers we detect early or the lives we save every day; we all focus on the one we missed. Yes, we are self-deprecating but our malpractice system, or lack thereof, reminds us of our failures.

In our school systems we are fighting for better student-to-teacher ratios so we can improve our elementary education and also prevent teacher burnout. We also have mandates as to how many patients each nurse can care for during any given shift. Yet a doctor's patient load is not a matter of concern. More teachers, more nursing staff are recruited as our patient loads increase, but to hire more physicians is the last resort of any administration. On an average night in the emergency department there is one doctor for seven to ten acutely ill patients. Just one.

Rising Patient Loads

The United States has fewer doctors per capita than comparable countries according to the Peterson-Kaiser Health System Tracker. Although the number of physicians continues to increase, the ratio is further widening in our country, as more people need medical care.[3]

Are more people requiring medical care because of our natural population growth? As our older generation ages and requires additional care, this should be offset by a younger, healthier generation needing less health care. That is how our Medicare program was built and thrived. However, while our elderly are living longer because of ever-improving medical care, our younger generation is requiring more medical treatments because of earlier onsets of chronic disease. Together, this combination is meaning more people needing medical care.

The health care system is placing ever more stress on physicians as our patient load is rising.

Because of technology, information is just a few clicks away for anyone, so few blindly trust medical advice. Now patients have demands that must be met. Modern-day medicine comes with expectations that the hospital is a technologically advanced place with highly skilled professionals expected to be infallible.

If you spend an afternoon in any doctor's office or hospital setting, chances are you're going to see the organizational chaos. Doctors, nurses, and administrative staff are in a frenzy and patients are hurried in and out of the exam rooms. There's minimal eye contact, because physicians must enter minutiae into electronic health records on laptops, rather than focusing on the patient.

No longer do we see one-on-one conversations with physicians. Now, you'll be talking, and the physician is typing. For every minute that you're talking, they're spending two minutes inputting information into your electronic chart. The only way for a physician to be efficient is to type while you talk. The reality is, by the time they see you, they are already behind and need to catch up on their notes so they don't spill over to the next day's workload.

An Increase in Expectations

On any given day you can find a story about a terminally ill patient filing for bankruptcy because of their medical bills. Or a diabetic skipping their insulin because they can't afford it. You may also find a story about a doctor who has killed himself.

As I was sipping my morning coffee one day, while the country continues to be obsessed with every politician's word, my eyes were drawn to the small title buried among the big headlines: "Junior doctor hangs himself at hospital where he had just started new job."

I didn't click on the article because I knew the story.

The medical profession relies on physicians to work extended hours, ignore their own signs of fatigue, and suppress any emotional toll that is the result of constantly witnessing tragedy. Physically, we function like highly trained athletes, but for us there's no Nike deal, private jet, or posh parties. Depression goes hand in hand with the medical profession, which is why doctors are far more likely to attempt and/or commit suicide than the general population—more than veterans, too.

Unfortunately, doctors know how to end their lives and have easier access to the means to do so.

During my internship, I was legally able to clock in eighty hours per week, but the reality was, we worked far more hours than that. We were offered rooms to sleep in at the hospital if we were too tired to drive home, but that would mean even more time away from our families. For me, I would call my mom or someone else during my drive home as a way to keep myself awake. I still do this. A friend of mine who was at the same stage of his training out in Los Angeles once got caught in traffic going home after a hellish thirty-seven-hour (clocked in as thirty hours) shift. He awoke to a police officer tapping on his window. He had pulled off the highway and parked under an overpass, and apparently had been asleep for several hours. When he was woken up by the police officer, of course it was assumed he was intoxicated. The impairment from exhaustion does resemble that of intoxication, but the officer allowed him to drive home after performing a full, humiliating field sobriety test on him. My friend was still in his work scrubs, and all of this played out in front of many onlookers on one of the busiest California highways. Exhausted. Embarrassed. Beat down. The same things that medical students, residents, and even many attending-level physicians feel daily. Day in and day out.

The rest of my day, following thirty-hour shifts, was a haze with the sound of my pager going off incessantly. I still feel a slight pang of PTSD-like panic when I walk through Target or some other department store and hear a sound that even remotely resembles the pager I had in my youth. Don't get me wrong, we're still at the beck and call of everyone, but now it's the sound of an email alert on our fancy smartphones. Perhaps less aurally offensive, but still the same intrusion.

As physicians we tend to form relationships with other physicians for many reasons, the most obvious being that we spend the majority of our lives in hospitals, so that is where we meet friends and lovers, and occasionally make enemies.

During a late shift one night, I wandered the halls of the hospital around 2:00 a.m. I had sat in a windowless dark room with limited human contact for nearly nineteen hours, and I was seeking a conversation. I was also seven months pregnant. I think it's funny how people say the hallways of a hospital are uncomfortable and "too sterile." When you work in a world of darkness, those blinding fluorescent lights of the hallway are quite welcoming. Although the rest of the hospital is eerily quiet at 2:00 a.m., the trauma bay is a segregated area where chaos remains in full effect, 24/7/365. Looking for human connection, I decided to sit down in the middle of the disarray and hope someone would have a few minutes for random conversation.

A new female doctor who had recently started at the hospital came by. Although I had heard about her from others and had spoken to her several times myself on the phone, this was my first in-person interaction with her. She sat down with me, and while the world spun around us, she and I became fast friends that late night (or early morning). She was slightly older than me, but our children were similar ages. She, too, was a type A personality, and she was also looking for the next mountain to climb.

Over a decade later, with three thousand miles between us, and the birth of a few more kids in the interim, our friendship stood strong. With most of my friends, although our in-person and even phone conversations are sporadic and short, the unspoken support is there. My friend was always the pillar of strength. A single mother and badass physician who conquered everything she encountered. She was invincible. Or so she had everyone believe.

During my own busy day at work, in and out of biopsies and delivering cancer diagnoses, I received a call from an unknown number. I usually decline such calls, but it was the perfect timing for catching me in between cases. I answered the phone before even thinking about rejecting the call. It was the supervisor at my friend's work asking me if I knew where she was. She had not shown up for her shift, which was scheduled to start thirty minutes earlier. Apparently my friend had put me down as her emergency contact at the time of her divorce. I can imagine that this would not alarm most people because it is quite often that someone misses a shift, a meeting, anything. But not doctors. We work through the flu, divorce, and even death.

I told her supervisor that she was sick and would check in soon. I didn't want to give any sort of indication that anything else was going on, because the long-term consequences could have been severe.

I called my friend. No answer. I texted her. Nothing. I called again. Voicemail. My nurse kept walking in to tell me my patient was waiting but my heart was beating too fast to hear her. Something was wrong. I had a missed call from my friend earlier in the week that I never returned. Did she need something? Why didn't I call her back? The constant fighting with her ex-husband was wearing, but she was staying on top of it. Her chief medical officer was filling her mind with profit-over-value discussions recently, and I knew it was getting to her, but she was stronger than all of that.

Thankfully I had her nanny's phone number saved in my phone. I called the nanny and asked her what the plan for the day was. She said that she had taken the children to school in the morning and was supposed to pick them up in two hours and bring them home and stay with them while their mom worked the late shift. I asked her if she had seen my friend that day, and she told me she had spoken to her through the bedroom door but hadn't seen her. I then asked her to go back to the house and check to see if she was home.

What felt like an hour later, but was really only eight minutes, the nanny called me from the garage and said my friend's car was there. The nanny rang the doorbell but no one answered. She didn't want to enter the house because she wasn't expected and didn't want to be intrusive. At that point I begged her to enter the house, but she refused. I called my friend's ex-husband, whom I had met. He thought I was overreacting, but I didn't really care. Thankfully he drove directly to her house and called me as he entered the house. He found her unconscious on her bed with empty bottles of pills and a note by her bedside apologizing to her children. I started screaming at him to check her pulse and call 911, but he was in shock and couldn't do anything. I hung up the phone and called 911 myself.

The toxicologist who treated her in the intensive care unit was a mutual friend of ours. It may be a big world, but it's a small medical community. With swift intervention her life was saved, but now came the part where we had to play cleanup to save her career, because doctors are not allowed to show weakness.

Perhaps that is why 300 to 400 doctors kill themselves every year, at a rate double that of the general population.[4]

Salary Shaming

Understandably, a lot of physicians burn out, and there are unique factors that contribute to it.

I completed four years of college, four years of medical school, five years of residency, and a year of fellowship. That's a lot of time and money. The next six years were devoted to trying to pay off my large, high-interest loans. It's not as though we come out of school suddenly at the top of the pay scale, either. We're on the lowest rung, and we must climb our way up the hierarchy of the medical system.

Medical school itself is arduous, with the long hours I've described, fierce competition, and constant examinations. It's amazing that the four-year graduation rate remains around 80 percent. Residencies and fellowships generally require working 80 hours a week, making 200 percent of the federal poverty level (Medscape 2019 average residency salary) for a family of four.

Yet the real stress comes when all the training is over and we become real doctors, only to learn we are getting paid less than those in our profession were making when we began our training. We have less time to spend with our patients. We are the main target of litigious people, and, now, the government has increased the administrative load and mindless computer work required to be reimbursed for our services.

All the altruism, the Hippocratic Oath, and the other reasons we wanted to be a doctor in the first place become overshadowed. It seems like every five minutes I must renew a certification or pay dues or some other bullshit fee. It is all a moneymaking scheme for various institutions and has nothing to do with health care or my ability to care for patients. Most recently, I had to take a multihour course on treating transgender patients and identifying sex trafficking victims. Was I reimbursed for this time spent away from my family outside of work hours? Absolutely not. We are rarely reimbursed for such required extra hours. If we want to maintain our medical licenses and jobs, we do what is required so that the institution can click on the box saying it is addressing the latest politically correct craze.

It boils down to this: medicine is a profession in which you are expected to be ever accommodating toward patients and administrators, infallible in judgment, and always benevolent. In most other lines of work, you can make mistakes. Physicians are not allowed mistakes. There are bad online reviews, egregious lawsuits, and the constant possibility of being dropped from the hospital system, losing your license, and your entire life's work altogether—there's no room for error.

When you say to a patient that they owe you money, they're shocked. They're offended you're charging them while they are *sick*! But patients forget that being sick is exactly why they need a doctor's services, and like any other kind of service—the plumber you call with a weekend emergency who comes right over to help you out—it costs money.

In California, the state publishes all physicians' salaries. Why should the public have access to that information? Physicians aren't government employees, so what is the benefit of this, other than to breed hostility? I see this as a gross invasion of privacy. Even more than that, if you found out that your physician makes more than you, would that alter your trust or confidence in them? Doctors are treated differently than other professionals because they are uniquely expected to do their job out of selflessness. But selflessness doesn't pay off the hundreds of thousands of dollars in medical school debt. It won't support their family, either.

It's a J-O-B

Just as in any other profession, a doctor performs a service and expects to get paid for it. Being a doctor is after all a j-o-b, and we all work for money.

Should surgeons be expected always to make sacrifices—rushing to the hospital in the midst of a special family occasion, for instance—to care for others, knowing the reimbursement for such lifesaving care may not cover their expenses for performing the surgery? Should the qualifications for being a doctor include not having a family or demands of their own? Are we approaching a time when the doctor will stop going in to care for patients because they are overworked, underpaid, and increasingly dissatisfied with their profession?

Physicians have lost the autonomy they once had. Physicians have become overwhelmed by the demands of electronic medical records, insurance formularies, regulatory requirements, administrative paperwork, and being constantly told to keep costs down while maintaining quality of care. Together, these demands contribute to an unprecedented level of burnout among medical professionals.

Third-Party Intrusions

After a workup and a treatment plan has been decided between you and the doctor, you are only halfway through the process. Now, the real challenge is to convince the profit-minded insurance company that the treatment prescribed is necessary: Otherwise, either you, the patient, must pay the costly price of the medication, or the doctor is forced to alter the treatment plan to accommodate the insurance company's preference. This glaring intrusion of the third-party insurer in the exam room further erodes the doctor-patient relationship.

Insurance companies have what's called a formulary, which is a list of medications that they will or will not cover. When a physician orders a test or treatment for a patient, the insurance company requires the patient and doctor to jump through bureaucratic hoops to get coverage for what was originally prescribed. It's very difficult to keep up with the formularies because they vary among insurance companies. Patients are upset when they go to the pharmacy only to find that the medicine their doctor prescribed isn't covered by the insurance company. Who should be held to task to know which medicines are covered on each formulary? Should there even be such a thing as a formulary? Why should a corporation trump the expertise of a physician regarding which medication a patient can have? The four years doctors spend in medical school learning biopharmaceutical physiology and then the three to nine years they commit to in residency and fellowships are apparently not enough.

Whether you have government-provided or private insurance, these plans determine what medication or treatment will be covered. When doctors work for the government, they are more inclined to prescribe the less costly, and potentially second-choice, drug because their payer is also their employer.

In the United States, our physicians still have the freedom to decide which treatment to prescribe. However, they are strong-armed by the insurance companies. Many doctors do not know the prices of medications. If they were more aware of the prices, they might be inclined to prescribe a less expensive yet equivalent medication or push more aggressively for nonpharmaceutical solutions (diet, exercise, over-the-counter remedies). Not all care denied by insurance companies is valuable or even necessary. But sometimes it is, and it can be expensive.

Perhaps it's the role of the pharmacist to discuss these nuances with the prescribing physician when the patient has been prescribed a costlier medication and there is a cheaper one available. If there is no such equivalent, then physicians should be able to prescribe the medication they believe is appropriate and the insurance company should cover it. Except there are actual laws heavily lobbied by pharmaceutical companies that prohibit this.

Networks and Payment Caps

In the same way that the AMA manipulated doctors as to which specialties maintain input, and how insurance companies have pharmaceutical formularies forcing prescribing trends, restrictive networks implemented by private insurers further regulate doctors. There are many doctors in your network, and your insurance company tells you which ones you can go to. That's because the insurance companies have essentially cut a deal with those doctors. They offer to pay them less to see their patients, but in exchange, the insurance company will funnel more patients to their offices. Thus, a doctor doesn't need to advertise because their name is listed in the available provider network and patients are limited to using them unless they want to pay out-of-pocket. This is why you spend less time with your doctors. They have to see more patients to make up for the loss in up-front revenue for each patient to be included in the insurance network.

Not every physician wants to do that, though—especially not those with established patients, successful medical outcomes, and good reputations. Often, these practices are classified as out-of-network because they have decided not to take part in the insurance companies' formulary. Commonly these include highly specialized doctors such as neurosurgeons, anesthesiologists, radiologists, et cetera; the professionals who have the most liability and underwent the lengthiest training (thus accruing more debt).

Let's say you have a child who's riding his bicycle. He gets hit by a car and smacks his head. You take him to the hospital, where the emergency room doctor sees him, and he gets a CT scan. The scan is read by the radiologist and the neurosurgeon is contacted because of a bleed in the brain. The brain surgeon comes in and performs brain surgery. There's also an anesthesiologist who is in charge of keeping the child alive and unconscious during surgery.

Typically, the only person in that scenario who is employed by the hospital is the ER doctor. Therefore, the hospital owns the lab work, the CT scan, and that doctor's fee. The specialty doctors are not employees, but rather make themselves available for covering emergencies at the facility. A brain surgeon at a single hospital would not perform a lot of cases. Therefore, it is more time- and cost-efficient for the surgeon to cover multiple hospitals. Since these doctors drop whatever they may be doing in their personal lives to tend to the emergency, they are less likely to accept reduced reimbursements for services rendered. In short, that means a brain surgeon is more likely to be out-of-network.

The brain surgeon then sends their bill to the insurance company. The insurance company refuses to pay the invoice because the physician is not in their network. This is where the concept of "surprise billing" comes into play. Insurers will either send a check for what they would pay for their in-network doctor or they may deny the claim altogether for the emergency lifesaving treatment.

If the insurer refuses to pay the billed price, it offers a devalued percentage of the charge and leaves a large balance on the patient's bill. It doesn't matter that the neurosurgeon came in at 1:00 a.m. or that the amount billed is the average of the services among other professionals in the area. Because the doctor is not allowed to bill the patient directly—a practice called "balance billing"—they must accept whatever the insurance company gives them and cannot request that the patient pay the residual unpaid invoice. For the record, the doctors don't want the patients to have to pay. This was an emergency situation and the patient should not be financially punished for getting care. Had this not been an emergency then the patient would have sought an in-network doctor. So, the fight is between the out-of-network doctors and the insurers.

The insurers want everyone to be under their network and take the reduced fee, because that's how insurance companies make a profit. How else will they pay for their lobbying efforts in the United States, spending over $445 million in 2019, based on public reports of campaign contributions?[5] These lobby giants convince government officials to legislate that the insurance companies should not have to pay out-of-network charges and should continue to allow narrow inclusion networks, which ultimately leads to less access for their patients and decreased reimbursement for the physicians. All of this is enshrouded under the headline of "surprise billing" legislation.

We see what being in-network does to our primary-care doctors, pediatricians, and many ob-gyns; the visits are truncated and many patients leave feeling dissatisfied with the interaction. Do you want this experience with the person charged with saving your life? Should the doctor ask the ambulance driver to sift through your wallet while you are crashing to make sure they are covered by your insurance company before deciding if they leave their bed in the middle of the night to save you? Or your child? Of course we don't, which is why these doctors often don't even know if their patient has health insurance until after they have intervened and cared for them. Insurance companies historically covered out-of-network physicians in emergency situations because they knew their value, but now, as they are being squeezed financially, one of the biggest moves has been to restrict a doctor's ability to be out-of-network.

FAIR Health is an independent, not-for-profit entity that was established to assist in the out-of-network debate. It promotes transparency in health care charges and also in insurance reimbursement rates based on a database of billions of billed medical services. From there, it provides a range of reported charges from varying geographic areas. This innovative process lays the groundwork for price transparency across the nation and, if used appropriately, would assist in lowering costs by encouraging price competition rather than price restricting. Unfortunately, the insurance lobby has pushed against using FAIR Health because it doesn't want to pay fair market value. Rather, it wants to force physicians to enter its network or replace them with someone who will accept the discounted fees.

Our physicians should be able to charge their set fee. If their charges are outliers on the FAIR Health data set, they will be pushed out of the market because someone is always willing to do something for less money; it's a truth we all live with. Although I would love to say these highly trained physicians are irreplaceable, the truth is, everyone is replaceable.

Rather than encouraging the FAIR Health method, state and even federal legislators are aligning with the insurance lobby and capping what physicians are able to charge based on Medicare rates, which themselves are low outliers on the FAIR Health range. The insurance companies are struggling to make profits under the Affordable Care Act, and their answer is simply to pay the doctors less and limit the number of doctors patients can seek care from.

It seems the only people who have the patients' backs are the doctors; yet they are overworked, short on time, and incentivized to hand out medications rather than to care for their patients.

Squeezing Out Specialty Doctors

Many projections have shown that we're going to continue to need tens of thousands more physicians to care for the American people. The shortfall is greatest within the surgical specialties. Specifically, neurosurgeons and transplant surgeons, who undergo the longest of all medical training, often an additional seven to ten years after graduating from medical school. A primary-care doctor, a pediatrician, and an emergency room doctor do an average of three to four years after school. During those years of residency training, they make a salary considered poverty-level in most states, if you break it down by the hours worked. During this time, they must begin to pay off their student loans, care for their families, and still make ends meet financially.

Other specialties like mine (radiology), my husband's (neurosurgery), ob-gyn, and others require double to triple the amount of training following medical school. That means incurring two to three times more debt and waiting two to three times as long to make a substantive salary.

So, it shouldn't be a surprise that specialists charge more for their services. Not only did they train longer and incur more debt, but specialists are also likely to be called away in the middle of the night or on a weekend to attend to high-risk situations with increased liability and less backup coverage.

With the Affordable Care Act and some of the proposed changes moving toward value-based medicine, the movement is to equalize pay across the board for physicians. A main objective is to increase reimbursements for primary-care doctors. When you have a fixed allotment of money that can go to health care professionals, any salary increase for primary-care doctors must come from somewhere. That's not to say they don't deserve an increase—they absolutely do—but it will come by way of a decrease in specialists' salaries. I have never heard of a pay cut as a solution to increase the quality of anything.

FREE TUITION

In 2018 NYU School of Medicine announced that it would offer free tuition to medical students. One hope is that this initiative will encourage more medical students to pursue careers as primary-care doctors, who earn less than specialists and thus have a harder time paying off their med school debts. That in turn would benefit underserved populations in the country where primary-care providers are urgently needed.

It's a noble idea, but it won't happen. The same ratio of students will go into specialty fields like surgery, radiology, and pathology, and the only difference will be that primary-care doctors will have less debt. In the short term, that's great, but will ultimately lead to lower doctor reimbursements and a stronger push toward socialized medicine.

An unintended consequence of NYU's decision—enabled, ironically, by a super-rich capitalist—*might* be to push the country toward socialized medicine.

The thing is, we *need* more primary-care doctors, so this is where Mr. Langone gets it right. Primary care is the front line in making America healthy again. They are point zero for individual health—by promoting healthy lifestyles, prevention education, and early cancer detection, they are vital in any step forward for us all. They deserve to be celebrated, and we need not only to incentivize medical students to consider primary care but to ensure underserved patients' access to them. But we can't do that at the detriment of our specialists, especially with potential long-term industry consequences.

Less Money, More Work

When it comes to physician job satisfaction, there are two main issues: feeling a sense of accomplishment in work, and the amount of work and frustration compared with income earned. We need to examine those two concerns in light of the ACA: nearly 20 million people obtained health insurance, and it happened overnight with Medicaid expansion. Higher demand for medical services by the newly insured requires a sizable workforce to meet that demand. Medicaid pays a mere 56 percent of what private health insurance pays in doctor reimbursements. (Medicare, on average, pays only 80 percent of what private health insurance pays.) These changes have allowed more people to get treatment, which is great, but this change was implemented with no preparation for doctors' increased workload and no concern for the paltry compensation doctors receive from government insurance.

The American health care workforce had faced shortages for decades, and this crisis was the straw that broke the camel's back. A system overload was inevitable—and it happened. As a result, there are long wait times to see overworked doctors. Moreover, people are less likely to see their doctor of choice, despite President Obama's infamous promise when pushing to pass the law.

Doctors quickly realized they couldn't handle the increased workload, and many had to stop taking certain insurances or stop seeing patients altogether. Pressures from the new reality under the ACA exacerbated burnout and dissatisfaction among many health care professionals, which contributed to the already developing physician shortage. Other doctors began taking on more patients to meet their expenses but then had to deal with the mountains of mandated paperwork.

Diminishing Role

Not only do insurance companies and legislators direct physicians on how to practice medicine, but now patients are directing their care, too. In the era of Doctor Google and online reviews, patients heavily scrutinize physicians' decisions based on incorrect information. Often, I will talk to a patient who starts out saying, "Well, I read on Google . . ." It takes every effort for me not to respond with, "Please do not confuse my medical degree with your Google search."

Sometimes I wonder why I'm even part of the conversation in the exam room. A few patients have already diagnosed themselves because a "fill in the blank" form online told them what they have, except it was completely wrong. Recently, a woman came to me with a mass in her breast that, after an ultrasound, I was able to confidently determine to be benign. Since it was the first time I was seeing her, and she was able to feel the mass, I wanted to follow up with her to document that it hadn't changed. Other than that, there was nothing else to be done. After a thorough discussion she appeared content with my recommendations, but the next day I received a call from her.

She'd spoken with her ob-gyn, who told her they wanted the mass biopsied. My role as the breast specialist was completely disregarded by the other physician, and now the patient herself was requesting a biopsy because her other doctor made her nervous about it. I had documented my entire report, providing my expert opinion that this situation did not warrant an invasive biopsy. I was now being strong-armed into ordering a procedure that I believed to be unnecessary.

For one thing, an unnecessary procedure increases the cost to the insurance company and the patient. For another, there is risk with every medical procedure. Although the risks are low, they are still present, such as chances of bleeding and infection. So, I put myself and the patient at risk for a potential complication because someone else demanded it. (The biopsy came back benign, for the record.) This is an everyday example of how our decisions as specialists are undermined, adding to the growing costs of unnecessary medical care.

It makes me wonder at times what my role really is if I'm not making decisions based on my decades of training and experience. Has my role transitioned into appeasing the patient—not to mention my employer, the insurance companies, and referring clinicians— at the expense of my own satisfaction? Am I really practicing medicine? It feels like I am perfecting my ability to placate others.

Defensive Medicine

In the United States, various states have passed tort reform laws limiting medical liability (the amount a physician can be sued for) in malpractice lawsuits. Yet there has been no tort reform legislation at the federal level. In certain countries there must be clear negligence on the part of the physician to result in any financial damages awarded to the patient, and such awards are subject to set limits. In America, some states have no limits on damages to be paid. Damages for "pain and suffering" are much higher in the United States than in other countries that award such damages. It is no wonder that American physicians must pay exorbitant premiums—tens of thousands of dollars—for malpractice insurance coverage.

Physicians are humans and make mistakes. As in every profession, there are a few outliers whose actions may be nefarious or downright negligent. Most medical errors are neither—they're just mistakes.

The lack of malpractice reform results in physicians practicing what some refer to as defensive medicine or, behind closed doors, cover-your-ass (CYA) medicine. When we're given only fifteen minutes to evaluate a patient, is it really so surprising mistakes are made? Naturally a physician does not want to miss a diagnosis, get the diagnosis wrong, or subject the patient to unnecessary testing and treatment. However, the fear of legal ramifications and lack of liability protection and time often lead to overutilization of diagnostic tests, procedures, and medications.

In my specialty—breast radiology—there are many physicians who have higher false-positive rates in their daily cancer screening. This means some call more exams abnormal when in actuality there is no cancer. Sometimes this is because of insufficient familiarity with what constitutes a benign finding versus a suspicious finding. At other times the physicians hesitate to let something go without working it up, despite their lengthy training and study of numerous academic studies supporting the benign etiology. Even if they know something is benign, some doctors are so afraid of malpractice lawsuits that instead of saying, "I'm 98 percent certain this is benign, so I'd like to see you back in six months to look again," they will recommend a biopsy to achieve 100 percent certainty in that moment. This results in an unnecessary and costly procedure, as well as undue anxiety and risk for the patient. Not to mention the mental fatigue of the back-and-forth communication.

No Rest for the Weary

As a rule, doctors rarely use leave/sick days appropriately for ourselves or family members. We have all gone into work when our children are ill or we ourselves are suffering from a sickness or injury. Years ago, prior to an anticipated snowstorm, I had the staff call every patient who was scheduled to come in on the day it was supposed to hit. I didn't want patients driving in dangerous conditions, and there is no level of nonemergent medicine that would warrant risking their safety. All the patients were rescheduled to come in a day earlier, double-booking my already full schedule. My staff and I stayed late that day, running around like madmen, but we were able to complete two days of work in one.

The next day, I woke up to a massive amount of snow that was blocking my doorway, driveway, and garage doors. There were trees down all over my yard, which had brought down live electrical lines, leaving the house without power. A massive fallen tree blocked the exit from my neighborhood. Thankfully, I was able to focus on my family and home, relieved to know that we had already cared for the patients originally scheduled that day. Now nobody, including my patients and myself, had to go out on treacherous roads.

Despite having no patients scheduled and my presence not being needed on site, my employer at the time docked me a vacation day. Mind you, I already had limited vacation time, so even one day felt like an assault on my family life. To take that day away was telling me, "We are punishing you for not leaving your children at home alone without power in a dangerous storm, even though you were proactive and managed to care for all of your patients ahead of schedule."

When I brought this to the administration's attention, I was told that it was the policy and it would not be altered despite my having made sure no appointment was canceled. Rather, I was told I should have stayed the night at the hospital. They would have provided a "bed in a box" for me even though there were no patients for me to care for.

Remember, I don't treat inpatients or acutely ill patients. Yet, regardless of my conscientious efforts always to provide high-quality care to my patients, my being physically present in the hospital in the absence of patients on the day of a dangerous storm was evidently of critical importance to my employer. Had this been the only time when I felt undervalued and disrespected, I would probably not have been so offended. However, our hours had recently been extended into evenings and weekends without so much as a conversation about it, and certainly without any immediate pay increase for our time. We were expected to go along with it. That mentality in the workplace can lead not only to a contentious environment, but it can exacerbate burnout. A colleague at the time told me one of our superiors had expressed the belief that there is no burnout for radiologists. In other words, appealing the extended hours was futile.

Physicians think they're above mental illness and addiction and will not succumb to it. But if their job turns into overwork, underappreciation, exhaustion, and work-life imbalance, alcohol and drugs might become a coping mechanism. For many, it does.

When Doctors Need Help

It's hard to get physicians to seek care, even when they know they need it. A good friend of mine, a high-functioning surgeon who I consider to be similar to myself in many ways, tried to take her own life. She had clear signs of bipolar disorder but on the high-functioning side of the spectrum. She was always motivated and had an incredible ability to multitask, which is what made her such a successful physician.

Her lows—the other side of a bipolar disorder—were few and far between. One day her lows took over, after the birth of her child. She manifested as severe postpartum depression. For the first time she wasn't the successful surgeon charging in and saving lives, so the change rocked her world and psyche. She spoke to a therapist but refused long-term follow up and medication because, as a physician, we tend to think we are smarter than any expert we see (I am not immune to this myself). That's the thing with doctors: we are quite stubborn, often to our own detriment. It was a tough time for her and her family.

Ultimately, she regained her normal high-functioning state. However, she wound up battling substance abuse over the next few years in an attempt to mask her fluctuating highs and lows. Several years later, she has now survived at least two overdoses. These were not cries for help; she wanted the pain of being out of control to go away.

Had she been on mood-stabilizing medicine at the first sign of her lows years ago, there's the potential we might have prevented these events and saved her reputation. When you're a physician who overdoses in a medical community, word gets around—even though we're supposed to be protected by patient privacy.

My friend is seeking help now, but probably not as much as she should. As much as we like to be perceived as superhuman or to play the savior, we are just human. We, too, struggle.

Even when dealing with an unsettling event or loss, doctors will rarely see a psychiatrist or use short-term medication to get them through because they fear experiencing discrimination for it. Every time we must be re-credentialed at a hospital or renew licensing, we are required to disclose whether we have been treated for mental illness. Those who do seek care will often pay cash, use fake names, or go to another town to get treatment. When they're asked mental health questions on licensing and other conventions, they'll lie about it. Even though it's illegal for employers to discriminate against someone on the basis of mental health, it happens. Unfortunately, I have seen this now with many colleagues, and the whispering continues.

Doctors witness pain, suffering, and death repeatedly. That alone can lead to depression. I deliver a cancer diagnosis nearly every day to seemingly healthy people. Add in the constantly increasing administrative burdens, loss of autonomy, and bureaucratic demands, and it's no wonder the suicide rate for doctors, as I have mentioned, is high. Doctors experience physical and emotional trauma every day yet are the least likely to seek help for it.

Reinforcements Aren't Coming

For the first time in decades, as of 2017 applications to medical schools were down. Of those who do apply for and attend medical school, a higher number have no intention of treating patients as their primary source of income. Instead, they plan to go into hospital administration with an MBA or malpractice law with a dual MD/JD—a career in which they can make millions—or start up their own medical device companies and maybe strike it rich there. Or they can use their credentials to become a CEO in the pharmaceutical industry, another highly lucrative career. All of this without having to deal with the bureaucratic bullshit that we underlings deal with.

NURSES ARE DECREASING, TOO

Shortages of doctors aren't the only concern: In a 2017 survey by the RNnetwork, almost half of the 600 nurses surveyed said they are considering leaving their field, and more than a quarter reported feeling overworked and burned out.[6] At some point, they're going to decide it's not worth it.

Even my choice to engage in advocacy, provide commentary on TV, and write a book is partly because of my own level of burnout. I realized quickly that I was able to reach more people advocating on their behalf through legislation and speaking directly to them via media or print. I had my first child at the age of eighteen and I've been trying to prove something to the world since that day. Now I'm settled into a career in which most of us are overworked, underpaid, and underappreciated. If my patients didn't show regard for my services, which often results in a sense of worth and accomplishment, I too might consider a change for my own benefit.

Like most physicians, I ask myself why I am tolerating the ancillary frustrations if my hard-earned opinion isn't even respected anymore. For most of us, it's for financial stability, but many of us also have high hopes for a return to a world where being a doctor was admirable. We still hope to be active contributors to the health of our nation.

Doctor shortages are already a reality. We find ourselves at a critical impasse: unless we shift our priorities to bringing autonomy and satisfaction back to physicians, and drastically reduce the amount of paperwork, third-party control, and self-inflicted disease, our physician shortage will continue to worsen. This will leave our most vulnerable patients without access to adequate care.

Chapter 9

WITH FREEDOM
COMES
RESPONSIBILITY

Every year 900,000 of our fellow Americans are dying too young, largely by means within their control that could have been altered.[1] It's astounding that there are still about 1,300 people dying per day in the United States from the effects of cigarette smoking, even after decades of literature telling us of smoking's dangers. As a physician, I lament losing even one patient to a preventable cause. It's staggering to know that hundreds of thousands of deaths each year are preventable. Yes, we have the right to live as we choose, but with rights come responsibilities. Our choices affect others. Just because something is a right doesn't mean it's free.

There are three broad groups of people as I see it: the healthy, the unlucky, and the obdurate. The unlucky are those who develop a disease they could not have prevented. The obdurate are those who develop a disease because their lifestyle choices involve known risks for the disease. Undoubtedly, there are many people who don't fit neatly in these categories, but let's paint in broad strokes for a minute. The problem with our system is that the unlucky and obdurate have been combined as one, and the healthy must subsidize that entire group. We are in a way mirroring the single-payer paradigm without having a single-payer system.

The difference is that health care in the United States, though more expensive than in other countries, was built on free-market competition. This has enabled us to have some of the most innovative treatments and diagnostic capabilities, not to mention the shortest wait times and most accessible system in the world. For this, the healthy are paying higher premiums for insurance coverage they may never utilize, and the obdurate are using health care services and insurance benefits without being held accountable for the choices that led them to need treatment.

In our politics, health care is just one of many issues on which we have a sharp partisan divide. Instead of tackling legitimate issues like our rising costs and overutilization of the system, politicians are looking for their next campaign slogans. Health care and the reforms needed to improve our system are much too complicated to be reduced to catchy headlines. Trying to do so only hurts those forced to navigate the system and our health care process overall.

Americans are desperate to put faith in their government to fix the health care system and are willing to jump on the next political campaign bandwagon "guaranteeing" it. Yet single-payer proposals lose their luster once the cost analysis is revealed.

Bernie Sanders's solution, a replacement of the current mix of private and government programs with a single government-run system, would cost between $30 trillion and $40 trillion over ten years. He claims the benefit of covering Americans outweighs the cost, but this plan also comes with as much as a 40 percent cut in compensation for physicians and health care providers.[2] Not only will this drive even more individual and small practices out of business, causing longer wait times for substandard care, but the government will begin rejecting treatments as non–cost effective.

Despite what politicians like Sanders, Warren, and others are saying, health care will never be "free." As a physician, I have devoted my professional life to caring for others. I graduated from medical school with $350,000 in debt and have worked hard ever since. Caring for patients is in many ways a reward in itself, but I cannot, nor should I be expected to, work for free. My colleagues can't work for free, hospitals can't provide services for free; drug makers can't bring new drugs to market for free.

It is utter foolishness to believe that implementation of a single-payer program in the United States will result in a happy (and healthier) America. Even if we wanted a single-payer system, we can't afford it—not with the amount of preventable disease and rampant overuse of our system. Why do we need to resort to this drastic measure anyway? Why can't we reform our system to simplify payment structures and reduce preventable diseases?

Socialism in America

A comical quote about socialism has been attributed to President Ronald Reagan: "Socialism only works in two places: heaven, where they don't need it, and hell, where they already have it." I'm convinced that most people who claim to support a socialistic health system have little understanding of what that would look like in America. They feel resentment toward those in power and cynicism about our nation, and they've been seduced by good political demagogues who promise them "free health care." Remember when a very well-known orator promised that with the implementation of the ACA everyone would be able to keep their doctor? How well did that promise work out?

When the responsibility of cost sharing is removed and everyone is provided with "free" insurance without maintaining individual accountability, there will ultimately be greater demand (and increased costs). This is what happened with implementation of the ACA and Medicaid expansion. Increase in demand and utilization without a corresponding increase in availability of care can lead to rationing and reduce access. That is the harsh reality if America adopts single-payer without drastic measures being taken to reduce preventative disease first.

Our political loyalties are blinding us to the practical problems with partisan utopian solutions. This blindness is hindering progress. We need to get out of our political bubbles and look at the larger problem: Americans have been making themselves sick, and individuals are not taking responsibility for their part in the problem. A new sense of responsibility for poor lifestyle choices would undoubtedly improve overall health, decrease the cost of health care across the country, and improve access and affordability for those who truly need medical services. Then and only then can we discuss the future of our health insurance paradigm. Besides, Americans have little idea what their health care even costs; no wonder they don't see a need to make a change.

Most people who have employer-sponsored plans don't have any real concept of how much their health care costs. Premiums are automatically taken out of their paycheck. They notice they have a $20 co-pay, or they know what their deductible is because they have to write that check, but they're not actually seeing how much it costs to go to the hospital or pay for their insurance coverage.

The Many Ways We Overpay

In the United States anyone can walk into (or be carried into) the emergency department and receive necessary emergency medical treatment, regardless of insurance status. This doesn't happen simply because of the altruistic nature of medical personnel, but because the Emergency Medical Treatment and Labor Act of 1986 (EMTALA) requires us to provide emergency services regardless of ability to pay. This extends to everyone who walks into the hospital, US citizen or not. Although this law was passed to protect the elderly and the poor, it has been applied to all patients. Meaning, undocumented immigrants and those who *are* financially able to pay for medical services yet choose not to have health insurance protection. EMTALA remains an unfunded mandate: people are entitled to receive emergency medical services regardless of economic and immigration status, but there are no designated federal funds to support this. The costs fall on hospitals, ED doctors, and the taxpayer. It is, therefore, a short-term solution with long-term consequences.

Anyone who has gone to the ED and waited for hours to be seen knows that emergency departments are crowded. Often, patients experiencing a mental health crisis will go to the emergency department because they don't have anywhere else to go. Anyone having an acute episode with nowhere else to turn should go to the emergency department so they don't hurt themselves or someone else. However, because of overcrowding, mental health patients may be discharged prematurely to clear space for other people. This is because of people who use the emergency room for nonemergencies. In fact, roughly 71 percent of emergency department visits could possibly have been treated adequately in an urgent care center or primary-care doctor's office. The emergency department is open 24/7, so people can go on their terms, whenever they want. If you go to the ED with a sprained ankle, you may be billed for $100, but your insurance company may be charged from $1,000 to $50,000 for your nonemergent workup. Patients are rarely charged the full amount, making the cost an abstraction and less of a deterrent than it would otherwise be. Studies have indicated that nonemergency treatment in emergency departments costs the system over $4 billion.[3] This is a major component of our unsustainable balance sheet.

Another concern pertaining to costs is the overuse of antibiotics, resulting in deadly antibiotic-resistant superbugs. When this happens, the more common, and less expensive, antibiotics must be retired and replaced with stronger, more expensive drugs. The average patient facing an antibiotic-resistant infection could expect a medical bill of between $18,000 and $29,000, totaling $20 billion in costs each year in the United States, according to a 2009 study by the Alliance for the Prudent Use of Antibiotics at Tufts University. In 2000, premature deaths, hospital stays, and lost wages related to antibiotic-resistant infections cost the United States $35 billion, Tufts researchers found.[4] Often these infections are acquired while a patient is in the hospital for another ailment.

This leads us to the problem of hospital-acquired infections and the role they play in our overall health care costs. Most infections that become clinically evident after forty-eight hours of hospitalization are considered hospital-acquired. Infections that occur after the patient is discharged from the hospital can be considered health care–associated if the organisms were acquired during the hospital stay. According to the CDC, on any given day about one in thirty-one hospital patients has at least one health care–associated infection. In September 2013 the CDC released a report estimating that overall annual direct medical costs of health care–associated infections ranged from $20 to $35 billion. Patients get big bills, insurance companies make big payouts, premiums rise, and the cycle goes on and on.[5]

Frivolous lawsuits are another factor driving up the costs. In the United States, we have more malpractice lawsuits than anywhere else in the world. That's not because our doctors are negligent or have subpar training—just the opposite, in fact. We are cared for by some of the most highly trained doctors in the world. The stark difference is that the United States is a litigious society. When something goes wrong or a treatment is not successful, some patients rush to place blame.

In addition to fears of malpractice suits, doctors are also becoming increasingly reliant on patient satisfaction surveys. In the vast majority of cases, people see their doctor because of a legitimate concern or complaint. However, a few come in for other reasons, such as wanting disability paperwork to get out of work for a mild ailment. The doctor recognizes that this is not a debilitating condition. Perhaps it may be as simple as knee pain that could be relieved by losing some weight or getting some physical therapy, but really no medical reason for the disability status. Physicians must be careful of what they say and whom they say it to because their online reputation is at stake. All too often, a patient will go online and write terrible reviews for the doctor or medical practice. If weight was brought up as the cause of an ailment, the patient might describe the doctor as insensitive or make accusations of discrimination. It is true that some doctors have biases, but I assure you they are few and far between, at least from my experience and encounters. What I see more often is that doctors are paralyzed by the fear of getting a bad online review. Once it's on the internet, it never goes away, and the ACA has tied doctor reimbursements to those reviews. Doctors are thus more likely now to meet patient demands, whether or not those demands have merit, because they find themselves in legal, reputational, and financial peril.

Covering Preexisting Conditions
Sets a Terrible Precedent

Our entire system is ineffective. It's ineffective for the physician, the patient, and the taxpayer, because it's reactive. People get sick and want to go in to have it fixed. We're not focusing on how to prevent people from getting sick in the first place, and the Affordable Care Act did little to change that focus. Its message was that you don't need to get yourself healthy. No matter what you have, it doesn't matter—we're covering it and we're paying for everything.

Although the ACA has created a demand for care, it has also created lengthy wait times to get appointments. In fact, in major cities wait times have increased by 30 percent since the implementation of the ACA. If it used to take eighteen days to get an appointment with your doctor, it now takes twenty-four days.[6] This highlights how the rationing effects are slowly trickling into the system and single-payer hasn't even been implemented yet.

In response to these factors, there's been an increase in concierge medicine, where you pay a doctor a flat fee per year for office visits and house calls. The price can vary from $80,000 a year for house calls and 24/7, 365-day availabilities to $500 a year for fewer services. Doctors in many other countries also use this model. Within their single-payer systems, you can pay a doctor a separate fee and be considered a "private" patient. This puts you ahead of those who have only government health insurance in the line waiting to be seen. Under the ACA and single-payer systems, those who can afford to will continue to maintain their elite privilege. The ACA may have promoted equal coverage but has actually separated the socioeconomic classes further.

We Should Not Label Behaviors That Lead to Healthy Outcomes "Privilege"

Americans believe that hard work pays off, and that everyone should have an equal opportunity to succeed. Of course, I would be remiss if I neglected to acknowledge the racial and gender inequality in our history that denied opportunity to so many. We have not and still do not always live up to our ideals. Today, it remains harder for some to advance in life because of the environment they were born into. Even so, there are people from all walks of life who have overcome extraordinary odds to reach success.

Why have we become reluctant to celebrate individual success stories, which could serve as models for others? Instead, self-made men and women are dismissed as being privileged.

I came from middle-class America. My parents met in college and lived with roommates during my childhood to make ends meet. They divorced before I can remember, and both worked multiple jobs to support themselves through college and graduate school, relying on federal and private student loans the entire course of their education. As they made their way up the academic ladder, I was just starting mine in the public-school system. Full days of honors classes, athletic activities, and part-time jobs were how I spent my adolescence. At least until I became pregnant between my junior and senior years of high school.

In a moment's time, I was marginalized, reduced to a teen pregnancy statistic. To say the next ten years of my life were easy would be laughable. However, without skipping a beat I gave birth to a healthy baby boy in the spring and started college at the local university that fall. Today, I live in the suburbs outside New York City with my family. I have become a highly specialized physician with a leadership position in the world's top cancer center. Yes, I did that. I was able to achieve success because of the tradition of meritocracy in the United States, and because of the freedom offered by our free-market capitalist system.

Are we to hide our accomplishments because many others have not achieved as much? Our country was founded on principles of freedom—including freedom to strive for success in the lives we have chosen; yet we now seem to be reversing this trend and denouncing those who followed through on their right to the pursuit of happiness.

Similarly, in health care, we're not supposed to praise the healthy for fear of offending the unhealthy. We're no longer supposed to point out to individuals that their own behaviors are the root of their ailments and financial burdens. Physicians are being criticized for being "prejudiced." It's evident in the emergence of the term "fat shaming." Obese patients are to be considered victims of their circumstances. Since the implementation of the Affordable Care Act, people who are healthier and doing well are being punished with higher premiums and higher deductibles to balance the losses incurred for the unhealthiest, who often pay less for their care. If we were to go to socialized medicine today, we would only further punish those with healthy lifestyles, who would bear even more of the health care cost burden.

Regardless of "privilege," the way our current system is set up, if you have healthy individual Y and unhealthy individual Z, Y will not be rewarded for healthy behaviors and Z will not be penalized for unhealthy behaviors. Z receives health insurance under the ACA without being held financially accountable for unhealthy behaviors, yet Y is penalized by paying more for the health insurance they rarely use (which technically is how health insurance is designed to work). Although some level of offset is expected in a normal situation, the cost associated with preventable disease is beyond acceptable. As a result, the middle class is paying for expensive plans that they cannot afford and may not even need.

Without a doubt, there are many medical conditions that we can't do anything to prevent. Regardless of the type of illness, every person deserves to be treated—I stand firmly by that. That's especially true for those who suffer from an affliction for which they had a genetic predisposition. I am afraid that, in our current system, it is not Z who is bearing the brunt of the burden, but Y, along with those whose diseases could not have been prevented, and we haven't accomplished much to fix it.

An Aging Population

Elderly Americans benefit from an array of costly medical treatments well into their golden years. Average life expectancy in this country is 78.6 years, but I sometimes find myself interpreting CT scans on people who are ninety-two and undergoing chemotherapy. As discussed earlier, Justice Ginsburg is a prime example of successful medical interventions for very old patients.

With some ailing elderly patients, however, we are prompted to question whether it makes sense to keep battling. Patients and friends ask me what sense it makes to put people in their late eighties and nineties through chemotherapy. Is there a point when we should say, "You've led a good life, it's time to enjoy your final years without being subjected to more medical intervention?"

It's a difficult and complex question without a clear answer, not just for doctors but for all of us. As a fellow human being, who am I to decide who does and does not get treatment? We treat everyone. But when we're running a ninety-two-year-old through the same grueling treatment as we would a forty-two-year old, it's natural to wonder, are we doing the right thing? At whose expense?

The Medicare system is fraught with problems for a few reasons.

Older people are receiving expensive care over the course of longer lives. When these patients are covered by Medicare, doctors and hospitals are reimbursed at much lower rates than they are for treating patients who are privately insured. As a result, doctors and hospitals overcharge those who are privately insured to off-set the deficit from the Medicare patients. We want seniors with Medicare coverage to get the best care, and doctors are required to provide it to them, but it's the privately insured population that indemnifies the losses from Medicare.

Private health insurance companies as a group are an unusual industry in that they decide how much they will pay regardless of the price that has been set. When you go to a flea market or swap meet, you expect to bargain. If you find an item for $6.00, you can say to the seller, "I'll give you $4.00 for it" (and the seller might come back with, "$5.00"). But you wouldn't do that in the grocery store. If a can of soup is marked at a dollar, you don't walk up to the register and offer 75 cents for it. Yet when a doctor submits a charge for evaluating a patient, let's say $100, the insurance company can then say, arbitrarily, "Well, I'm only paying you $80." They can make that decision, flea-market style. Doctors and hospitals can fight these decisions (they can bargain), but much of the time they go along with it because the fight isn't worth the time and effort. Yet, whatever fraction of the charge the private insurance reimburses, for the most part that amount still exceeds what the government-program reimbursement would be.

The federal program also incorporated private insurance plans into Medicare to help cover additional "hidden" costs for elderly patients, like their expensive medications. Thus the private insurers are paying more, and younger, healthier people are paying higher premiums, to counter the payout for the elderly. Medicare was developed so that seniors would be guaranteed health insurance, with costs subsidized by their prior employment contributions, federal dollars, and some supplementation from those privately insured. The law was passed at a time when life expectancy was shorter and medical care not as advanced, so the amount of care received after the age of retirement was less than the amount received today. In addition, Medicare is not means-tested—it is available for anyone regardless of income or assets. The Medicare system is now financially stressed to an alarming degree. We are quickly approaching the point where we may have to substitute the Medicare model our seniors are accustomed to with the Medicaid model. This is why the slogan "Medicare for All" is so comical. We will not be able to afford high-priced Medicare coverage to our elderly, let alone all Americans, if we do not take action to decrease the cost of care.

Just look at what is occurring across the Atlantic Ocean. In the United Kingdom, physicians are government employees, and therefore the government makes decisions as to who gets treated and by which method. This government power has led to dramatic cases like those of the infants Charlie Gard and Alfie Evans, whom the NHS removed from life support against the wishes of their parents. Thankfully, in the United States patients and their families, not the government, make such choices. I would not want to be in a situation where, as a doctor, I must consult with government officials on which patients will or will not receive treatment based on budget concerns.

Other Health Systems

Canada

Far-left liberals often remind us that we should learn from the rest of the world's health systems, but the lessons we learn may not be the ones they wish us to heed. Canada's single-payer system is an outline of Bernie Sanders's Medicare for All plan yet does not cover everything his plan promises to. Canada incorporates some private insurers within its system. People pay extra for medications, dental care, and ambulance transport. Canadians also have the choice of purchasing private insurance for medical care that is otherwise covered under the nationally funded system.

Contrary to a lot of talk, Canadian health care is far from free, and it comes with high taxes and great inconvenience. To see a specialist, you might wait up to thirty-five weeks, when in the United States it's closer to thirty-five days. You'll be treated immediately for something acute, like a heart attack, but chronic conditions and testing come with significant wait times.

Canadians who can afford it will come to the United States for medical services so they can bypass the long waits in their own country. The Fraser Institute estimated that over 63,000 Canadians traveled abroad for medical care in 2016. We know the reason they're coming is not that our prices are lower, it's that they are given more efficient access to exemplary medical service.[7]

The United Kingdom

The National Health Service is a government-funded system under which health care services are free at the point of service. In recent years concerns have been mounting that the NHS is becoming financially unsustainable, and patients routinely voice dissatisfaction with wait times and quality of care.

In 2018 the British Red Cross said that the country is nearing a national health crisis because of a severe shortage of physicians. The General Medical Council (GMC), a doctors' regulatory group, warned that the problem had become critical, threatening patient safety. Faced with too many patients, a stifling bureaucracy, and forced to perform tasks beyond their expertise, doctors were cutting corners in ways that are harmful to patients. The GMC warned that "the UK is running out of time to prevent a significant decline in workforce numbers, which risks patient safety" and that "the medical profession is at the brink of a breaking point in trying to maintain standards and deliver good patient care." The GMC's survey of 2,600 UK doctors found that one in five was considering cutting back to part-time or seeking work abroad.[8]

In a drastic money-saving move, the NHS has begun restricting surgeries that the NHS England medical director described as "useless." These include spine surgery for chronic low back pain, nonemergency gallbladder removal, and hernia repair. The NHS has told patients they have a responsibility not to request surgery that "does no good." Don't you love when a government decides what is good?[9]

In some parts of the UK, the NHS has begun rationing care for patients who are obese or who smoke. Knee and hip surgeries, for example, will be denied for up to a year for those patients. Officials warned that, because of the NHS "funding crisis," this could be just the beginning of a wider use of rationing.[10]

Now, I'm not saying that I necessarily disagree with the notion of giving patients an incentive to quit smoking or lose weight, at which point they can get their surgeries. The UK can't afford the procedures and don't have enough doctors to perform them, so they mask these deficiencies with the excuse that it's good for the patient. The real reason is that they don't have the supply to keep up with the demand. Regardless of the reason for the NHS rationing, this concept would be very difficult for Americans to wrap their heads around.

The situation in the UK should serve as a wakeup call to Americans who criticize our system. Yes, it is costly, yes, it is redundant, but at least we excel in terms of access, quality of care, and patient choice. At some point we will have a Democratic president with a Democratic majority in Congress, as with President Obama when the ACA was passed. Will single-payer be the next step? When that fails, what will be their next solution?

Iceland

Iceland is another country with a universal health care system, paid for through taxes and delivered by the Ministry of Welfare. The system includes some cost sharing: for medication to treat serious illnesses, roughly 75 percent of the cost is reimbursed, while patients generally pay for antibiotics. The European Observatory on Health Systems and Policies reports that Iceland has seen a 76 percent increase in out-of-pocket costs from 1995 to 2010. This rise has led to increased taxes and some other less traditional cost-saving methods.[11]

In recent years, Iceland has gotten press for its extremely low rate of Down syndrome in the population. This is not due to a lower incidence of the genetic mutation that causes Down syndrome, but because of a higher rate of abortion when prenatal testing indicates the presence of the mutation. In such situations, close to 100 percent of Icelandic women choose to terminate their pregnancy.

In the United States, the termination rate for Down syndrome is about 67 percent. That's a big difference, and there are multiple reasons for it. The Icelandic government mandates that, when a woman is found to be carrying a fetus with the genetic mutation, she is to be counseled on the option to abort the fetus and the difficulty of raising a child with disabilities.

What's the impetus behind that mandate? In large part it has to do with the high cost of care that babies born with Down syndrome will need. From birth, through childhood, and into adulthood, they will have chronic health issues and require more care, which necessitates more government assistance. Reducing the number of people with Down syndrome in the population decreases the overall price tag for their health care.

If our costs continue to soar in the United States, is it so far-fetched to assume Americans, too, will be urgently counseled to terminate pregnancies, knowing that our stressed system won't be able to care for disabled children? Do we want the government to have that power over us? If we don't take charge of reducing some of our preventable disease in order to reduce the burden of the overall budget, future generations may face a situation like the one in Iceland. Perhaps that's an extreme example from a tiny country, but we can't hide our heads in the sand about the problems other countries are facing.

Just Say "No"

While I don't believe doctors should refuse care, I do think insurance companies should refuse to pay for some or all services in certain situations. I also believe physicians should be allowed to require payment up front in nonemergent circumstances to ensure adequate compensation for services rendered. We shouldn't insist that insurance companies pay for elective surgery for patients whose health is compromised by their own unhealthy behaviors. Such patients are at increased risk of complications, which ultimately costs the insurer even more money.

People can be given the option—if you don't want to quit smoking and are willing to pay a higher premium and accept responsibility for complications related to smoking, you can make that choice. I would prefer that the patient make that choice rather than the government. Americans are not one-size-fits-all and neither are our health care needs.

If we want to change our broken system, failing single-payer systems are not the model. We can lower costs—that part will be easy—but the difficulty will be maintaining quality and access to care. The only way to lower costs and preserve quality or even improve quality is to lessen demand.

If we get rid of redundancy and overutilization—the inefficiencies of our system—as well as lessen preventable illnesses, we'll have markedly lower costs and thus more funds to subsidize those who cannot afford health care. We will also put more dollars in Americans' pockets.

The Solution

I support a strong privatized health industry intertwined with equally robust government health services. However, we must eliminate inefficiencies of government programs, including the Veterans Administration system, the Indian Health Service, Medicaid, and even Medicare.

The VA is an embarrassment and utter disservice to Americans who have served our country. It's plagued with antiquated record keeping, dangerously long wait times for appointments and treatments, lower physician-to-patient ratios, and a constant revolving door of employees because of less than competitive reimbursements and poor work conditions. The deterioration of VA health care is a consequence of many systemic failures. It serves as a stark example, here in the United States, of how government-run medical care can have not just mediocre but terrible outcomes for patients.

It is time for us all to roll up our sleeves and get to work on making a change and improving our private health system. There are steps we can take, regardless of our politics or positions on the health care issue, to lessen the financial burden on our system.

Chapter 10

THE AMERICAN
HEALTH SYSTEM

The privatization of America's health system did not happen overnight. If there is to be any attempt made at fixing a broken system, then it would behoove us to understand how it became the way it is today. Back in the early 1900s, health care essentially boiled down to which crazy cure we preferred in the moment, including mercury rubs and brain lobotomies. Needless to say, unless something drastic was being tried, the cost of routine health care was not an issue for most of the population. As the twentieth century progressed, and as technology, including anesthesia and radiology, evolved, the associated cost of care subsequently increased. People were still in favor of paying for catastrophic care, but the concepts of preventative care and long-term disease management had not been cemented.

No one had worked out the solution to supplying costlier innovation yet keeping them affordable to patients. So, Baylor Hospital in Texas started looking for a way to get people to pay for health care the same way they paid for other necessities, such as a mortgage: a fraction of the cost each month.

With the primary mission of ensuring hospitals were paid for providing care to sick people, BlueCross BlueShield of Texas was born. The Baylor-derived company originally functioned as a nonprofit, starting off small by offering a barter system to public-school teachers. The arrangement allowed teachers to pay fifty cents a month in exchange for covering hospital costs at Baylor if they were needed.

The timing was perfect for the inception of BlueCross Blue-Shield because as the Great Depression hit, the hospital patient loads dwindled. People could barely afford sugar and bread; how could they be expected to pay for medical services? Since medical technology was still evolving and the costs to produce them were rising, Baylor's insurance idea became quite popular; thus thrusting forward the concept and opportunity of private health insurance.

Initially, the approach was that the insurance company would pay all the charges, regardless of cost. However, as the medical community was trying to increase utilization of the health system, a nationwide debate grew over how to manage the rising costs. In 1926 at the annual meeting, one of the main questions on the agenda for the American Medical Association was how to raise demand for medical services during this calamitous time.

As the end of the Depression grew near, the 1935 National Labor Relations Act was passed to protect the general welfare of workers and avoid unnecessary obstruction of economic commerce by strikes and other forms of industrial unrest. This law became the catalyst that caused private health insurance to grow. Blue-Cross BlueShield companies offered employer-based discounted plans to help in employment negotiations and allow more working Americans to access the health system. By World War II, what had started as BlueCross BlueShield expanded into an entire industry, with many different companies, price controls, and large government tax incentives.

The rest is history.

Hospital costs continued to rise under an inflationary economy. After a few decades of unchecked rising health care prices, insurance companies formed health maintenance organization (HMO) plans to encourage price competition and improve quality of care. This was done by creating a network of doctors willing to be compensated lower amounts in return for having the insurance company deliver patients. However, the cost-control methods created a backlash among patients because this move created financial incentives to deny patients care and restricted access through formularies.

Thus, preferred provider organization (PPO) plans were developed because patients demanded more choice of who they went to for medical services, rather than the limited networks of a less-expensive HMO plan. For many, quality of care and immediate service were more appealing than affordability. This concept has been and continues to be a staple of the American health care system and sets us apart from nations with socialized medicine. However, once PPOs were available, insurance companies needed to find another way to limit the cost of care.

One of the most controversial methods to save on hospital charges was to send the mothers of newborns home after a day in the hospital, with insurers refusing to pay for additional days following an uncomplicated delivery. Congress intervened in 1990, passing legislation mandating coverage for at least forty-eight hours after delivery. The length of stay needed following birth varies widely; some women are able to leave within hours, whereas some require longer times in the hospital. Regardless, the physician and new mother should be making decisions about how long to stay, not the insurance company. Where health care deviates from the normal market, the payer *should* have a stake in the game to decrease overutilization. Ultimately, though, patient care and safety are best left up to the doctor, not necessarily the payer.

We very much made a bet on private insurers as the way to

manage costs, and the consequences are large, restrictive networks. Not to mention high insurance premiums and out-of-pocket costs. We have allowed the insurance companies to become Goliaths towering over the Davids of doctors and patients. The smaller medical practices are being bought out by the larger systems because they cannot compete in the market anymore. As a result, the patients are herded like cattle into the insurance networks without the ability to decide where or from whom they receive their care. We are now emulating a government-run system in a "free" market environment.

Misplaced Focus

The maintenance of a free market in US health care has received an enormous amount of criticism because of the perceived mantra of profit without relation to value. It also failed to restrain costs. In a private report leaked to news outlets in the spring of 2018, an analyst from Goldman Sachs cautioned against investments in pharmaceutical or biotechnology companies focusing on medical cures. Simply explained, if profit is the goal, then a product aimed to cure will eradicate its own demand. This simple analysis fueled every conspiracy theory against privatized health care.

Though the report makes for bad optics, we have to keep in mind that this was the viewpoint of an investment company, and not that of doctors, hospitals, or even pharmaceutical companies. Much innovation comes from a private system with numerous investors, but it's something of an externality to acknowledge the motivation to make money.

Because investors are more inclined to seek the projects that will have maximum return, Congress passed the Orphan Drug Act (ODA) in 1983 to encourage increased development of drugs treating rare diseases such as ALS, Tourette's syndrome, Huntington's disease, and muscular dystrophy. Rare diseases are illnesses affecting less than 200,000 people; the definition also applied to diseases affecting more than that number if there was no commercial viability for the treatment (meaning the cost of development would exceed US sales revenue). For this, the drug companies were offered large tax breaks on expenditures as well as grants and seven-year market exclusivity. As a result, many more orphan drugs were introduced (10 prior to the ODA, now more than 450).

My sister and I both benefit from this legislation. We live with autoimmune diseases that are treated by medications with orphan drug classifications. Thankfully, as these drugs come with a hefty price tag, we are both covered by employer-sponsored health insurance. Through an HSA account, I pay my out-of-pocket portion of the drug with tax-free dollars, and my sister uses the coupon program based on financial need.

Although many lives are being improved and even saved by the ODA, the controversy surrounding this legislation is driven by the health insurance industry, which has declared that pharmaceutical companies are gaming the system to maximize profits. Unfortunately, some drug companies have indeed gamed the system by taking existing medications and obtaining orphan status for them for other uses.

Scott Gottlieb, a physician appointed by President Trump to serve as FDA commissioner, who is now retired, addressed the concerns of the ODA in an opinion piece in 2018. He acknowledged the lives saved and immense progress made as a result of the legislation. However, he criticized pharmaceutical companies for maximizing their profits on these drugs. Many of the orphan drugs that came on the market were priced exceedingly high; but since they had market exclusivity, there was no market competition or price caps limiting what they could charge. Although the

ODA is still under scrutiny and likely to be the topic of future debates, under the Trump tax reform, the tax breaks for manufacturers of orphan drugs have already been reduced from 50 percent to 25 percent.

Of course, most Americans' illnesses aren't caused by a collection of rare diseases. As a nation we are suffering from a collection of common diseases, like cardiovascular disease, obesity, diabetes, and various cancers. Few resources are being invested in new treatments for common ailments. Behavioral changes, weight loss, exercise, and a healthy diet, don't receive enough emphasis, even though contemporary research confirms how important they are in preventing disease. True, there's a good deal of profit being made in the wellness market—wearable tech, fad diets—but there isn't much more wellness to show for it.

It's not hard to see why there has been less focus on risk prevention: profitability. The disease treatment landscape is based on the premise that health care is a service industry, no longer delivery of expertise and miracle treatments. The industry exists to create a profit, and people changing their lifestyles for the better decreases those profits. So, what incentive do people in the business have for promoting healthy diet and exercise? *None.* This attitude has contributed to decades' worth of continued self-destructive behaviors and the rising prevalence of chronic, yet preventable, diseases. This is also the foundation for criticism of a privatized health system.

Cart before the Horse

We have healthy young individuals, healthy older individuals, individuals who are sick because of poor lifestyle, and individuals who have unavoidable conditions. Without a doubt, we want to take care of each group. The question remains, should private health insurance be responsible uniformly for all of the above populations? The people who make poor behavior choices and get sick because of them are driving up costs for everyone else. We are putting the cart before the horse, and it's causing a major pileup.

Where did we go wrong and where did this lack of accountability come from? The Affordable Care Act, designed to treat everyone equally, sounded to many like a great reform. Yet the ACA cemented a sense of entitlement regarding insurance coverage and care, regardless of health status. Coverage for preexisting conditions is still the most popular provision under the ACA, but it has destroyed the incentive for people to make modifications to better their health.

The word "insurance" has lost its meaning. It used to mean being financially protected if you got sick or injured—you bought insurance before you got sick. Now that preexisting conditions must be covered, insurance means getting paid after the fact. The burden on the entire insurance system has resulted in higher premiums and deductibles for everyone. We're still going about this from the wrong end, when what we need to do is urge people to lead healthier lifestyles to begin with.

Senator Chuck Schumer commented in April 2019 that Trump's attempt to dismantle the ACA would force women to pay more for their health insurance and deny cancer patients treatment. This sort of bombastic statement is common from both sides of the aisle, intended to create hysteria.

Here's the truth. The Affordable Care Act enacted rules that prohibited health insurance companies from charging higher premiums for women. As a woman, I hate to break it to everyone, but data from the National Institutes of Health confirm that per-capita lifetime medical expenditures for women are nearly $100,000 more than for men. It's not gender discrimination for insurance companies to charge women more, it's math. The emotional rhetoric helps no one.

As for Schumer's claim about cancer, when an insured person is diagnosed with cancer, treatment has historically been covered. If the diagnosis is received prior to the patient's obtaining insurance, or the patient must switch insurance policies while receiving treatment, this is where the lapse in financial coverage can occur. No insurance company wants to take responsibility for covering the costly illness, leaving patients in a very difficult position. Because of this subset of patients, the ACA mandated that insurance companies pay for each illness regardless of time of diagnosis, muddying the entire concept of what insurance was designed for. But there was an alternative: the law could have mandated short-term plans that use high-risk pool funding to cover the costs for these patients. Yet politicians on the left would have you think that by changing the preexisting condition mandate within the ACA you would destroy coverage for patients with cancer.

The truth is, both parties have long supported covering preexisting conditions in some way, and anyone telling people otherwise is using politically motivated scare tactics. Every plan proposed by congressional Republicans over the last several years included some form of coverage of preexisting conditions. The difference with the ACA is that it took preexisting condition coverage one step further. Not only must insurance companies cover the cost of the disease acquired prior to coverage, but they can't charge the person any more for it. The individual mandate was supposed to make sure people didn't take advantage of the preexisting condition provision by waiting to get sick or injured and then buying insurance the next day. Clearly, that aspect of the ACA wasn't received well, nor did it accomplish its goal.

Who can forget when President Obama said, "If you like the plan you have, you can keep it. If you like the doctor you have, you can keep your doctor, too. The only change you'll see is falling costs as our reforms take hold." In fact, he made variations of this same declaration to the public at least thirty-seven times between inauguration and when the law was enacted.[1] I think everyone missed the fine print in this false promise. After public outcry Obama had to clarify his promise: "Now, if you had one of these plans before the Affordable Care Act came into law and you really liked that plan, what we said was you can keep it *if it hasn't changed since the law passed*."[2] Funny enough, that little caveat was never mentioned before.

So why did people start losing their health insurance plans? By 2014, just a few years after the ACA was enacted, over 5 million people had their existing individual market plans canceled. What Obama was referring to when he said you could keep your plans was the grandfathered plans that existed prior to the ACA. These plans were mainly employer-based and could continue without offering the essential health benefits as long as they did not deviate from their pre-ACA design. The benefit to the insurer for maintaining grandfather status is that it is not subject to the ACA cost-sharing limits and did not need to meet the essential benefits status, thus reducing cost per individual. However, although these plans did not need to conform to all ACA requirements, they did have to adopt many of its administrative headaches in addition to the ban on preexisting exclusions, lifetime/annual dollar caps, and covering dependent children up to twenty-six years old. The ACA itself changed insurance policies, which instantly refuted Obama's promise to Americans. The ACA caused the premiums to rise to cover these extraneous additions, forcing many companies out of the market.

When President Trump first entered office, he used an executive order to direct federal agencies to gather information as to why individual plans had difficulty maintaining grandfather status and what kept people in grandfathered vs. non-grandfathered health plans. The results supported the argument that the agencies should lessen the 2015 regulations on grandfathered coverage. In April 2019 the Trump administration extended existing grandfathered plans through 2020 to keep these popular, less-expensive options while longer-term solutions are explored.

Possible alternatives to ACA provisions include a combination of grandfathered plans, expanding use of HSA funds for out-of-pocket costs, and increasing the duration of short-term health plans from three to twelve months. Regardless of the specific plan, cost sharing should be a fundamental component to the policies.

Cost Sharing

Let me tell you why cost sharing is a good thing.

Cost sharing means the insured and the insurer are sharing the cost of medical care. Cost sharing outlays for the insured include out-of-pocket costs in the form of deductibles, co-pays, and co-insurance. Not only does cost sharing help keep premium rates manageable, it also prevents overutilization of health services by deterring unnecessary use. The ACA eliminated cost sharing for many services, including cancer screening. The benefit of this was an increase in overall cancer screenings. However, this contributed to rising costs of care. When the cost sharing was removed from certain services, the price of premiums and other services rose to compensate for the loss.

In 2014 President Obama signed into law HR 4302, whose main provisions had to do with Medicare but which also increased annual deductible limits for group plans. In 2015 the average deductible for self-coverage was $6600 ($13,200 per family); in 2019 rose to $7900 ($15,800 per family.) To balance the increase in cost for the sick, healthier individuals were not only paying higher premiums for their coverage, but they were paying more out-of-pocket costs than ever before when they did not even require medical care. The problem was that the ACA did not concomitantly lessen restrictions on tax-free funds in Health Savings Accounts (HSA) to help with the out-of-pocket expenses.

The trick here is to find the sweet spot of cost sharing through tax-free HSA accounts and third-party coverage. Emergency situations such as a stroke, heart attack, or a broken leg are prime examples of why we have insurance. These are crises that render us unable to use discretion when seeking acute medical care. When physically or mentally incapacitated, we cannot make such decisions but rely on the professionals to make rational decisions for us. Balance-billing laws prohibit the doctors who care for patients from billing them for emergency care if they are not in the restrictive insurance networks, which is to say, if they are out-of-network.

Back to the Basics

People should not go bankrupt because they were unable to price shop or determine network status during an emergency situation. What about non-urgent health care needs, especially preventive care? Recommendations vary for cancer screenings, routine checkups, and most diagnostic imaging. I have my own opinions, but so do many other doctors. Because of this variability, it is important for the individual patient to make decisions based on their own risk-benefit analysis of this type of medical care.

Rather than a one-size-fits-all approach, we are moving toward precision medicine, in which treatment options are tailored to an individual. This is promising because it encourages not only individual decision making but individual cost sharing. Including the cost in the equation gives a more accurate analysis of risk vs. benefit. If the sole financial responsibility is on the third-party payer, then there are no safeguards to ensure financially sound decisions are being made. It is much easier to gamble in Vegas if you are using someone else's ATM card. The moment your own paycheck is at stake, you may prefer a more conservative approach and only go "all in" when you have aces in the hole.

Imagine if we created a system in which the insurance companies would cover our catastrophic illnesses, such as a cancer diagnosis or a ruptured brain aneurysm, and as individuals we took steps to prevent those illnesses from occurring. We could re-create the ideal health insurance environment, where patients have stake in the game. For the nonemergent scenarios, the insurance company would provide a lump sum of money, and the patient would be responsible for determining where they go for their care. With a lump sum coupled with tax-free HSA accounts, people could budget the necessary with the unnecessary. This scenario would demand providing price transparency, improved HSA user ability, and low-cost alternative plans; all staples of most Republican health care proposals. I dare to take it one step further.

In defiance of naysayers (it is easy to sound like the bad guy here), I challenge America not only to support these types of reforms but to look in the mirror and see what more can be done.

Routine wellness checks and vaccinations are essential to keeping Americans as healthy as possible. As we age, we need to add cancer screenings like mammograms and colonoscopies to our routine. People need to work with their doctors to determine the most appropriate and beneficial schedule for them to maintain. They should also choose the doctor and location from which they want to receive care, based on price and satisfaction, not because their insurance company is directing them. This is where price transparency comes into play. Giving patients the freedom to choose their medical practitioners and sites where they receive care rather than forcing them into a provider network will encourage market competition. It will not only maintain prices but spur improvement in quality and patient satisfaction. The patients will reward themselves by budgeting and will have a surplus in their HSA accounts. Remove the restrictions associated with the tax-free funds and allow people to use them for other necessities such as toothpaste, menstrual products, and even gym memberships. The patients who are responsible for saving money while also utilizing preventive care should be rewarded for their efforts.

The insurer could further reward them for meeting certain wellness metrics, acknowledging their efforts to reduce their chances of developing disease. Say you go to your primary-care doctor and discover you have high cholesterol. After discussing methods of lowering cholesterol, whether through diet and exercise alone or in combination with medicine, you decide on a plan. At the next appointment, if the test reveals you have effectively lowered your cholesterol (therefore drastically lowering your risk of developing heart attack, stroke, dementia, and kidney disease), you receive a reduction in your insurance premium or a reduction in your co-pays contingent on maintaining it. Why are people opposed to positive reinforcement when it comes to our health?

The ACA attempted to introduce value-based medicine but got it backward. According to the theory behind the ACA, the incentive for patients to be healthier was to jeopardize payments for doctors and hospitals if successful results are not achieved. Although this approach might help certain practitioners and sites improve their techniques, I would venture to say a larger benefit would be achieved if the patient was also incentivized to get healthier. Though well-intentioned, the law took a system already overburdened with administrative and regulatory tasks and made it worse. The new initiative to prove "value" (whatever that means) in services further impedes delivery of patient care.

The ACA uses excessive regulation to try to get better health outcomes. The overwhelming transition to bundled payments, value-based reimbursements, and infinite box "clicking" on EMRs has left our physicians chasing their payments rather than focusing on patient wellness. Increased regulation does not, in fact, lead to improved patient care. I am not saying that the system should go back entirely to fee-for-service, where doctors were paid for each service provided whether or not it worked. However, the concept of value-based care and what we define as value should be further explored.

Sick individuals will need medication, hospitalization, and frequent doctor visits, all of which are expensive. We do not want to punish those who are already sick by barring them from coverage or burdening them with costly medical bills. However, we must reward people for better choices that lessen the risk of disease and subsequently lower their cost of care so that more resources can be used on the infirm. Living healthier lives means lessening the cost of individual care. The insurance company can cover more and charge less for others with expensive medical needs. The savings help us all, providing value to our overall system.

Bottom line: We want to take care of everyone, but we need to do it in smarter ways.

The Stick *and* the Carrot

Workplace health incentive plans were originally created to motivate employees toward higher wellness achievement. Incentive plans that reward employees for reaching preestablished goals provide encouragement and give them something to aim for. The advantage to the employer is increased levels of productivity—and, in turn, increased productivity and wellness also become an advantage for workers.

Although the concept of work-wellness programs seem positive and show some benefit, they are not very good at improving the overall health of employees, nor do they lower the overall cost of care.[3] The findings were published as a working paper at the National Bureau of Economic Research. In fact, employees with the highest medical costs are actually the *least* likely to participate.[4] The only uptick in participation in wellness programs, albeit minor, was seen when financial incentives were offered for participation. The bottom line is incentives work, and not costly "feel good" programs. Yet companies continue to pour money into them. The wellness industry in the United States is estimated to surpass $179 billion in 2020,[5] with $8 billion alone in workplace wellness programs.[6] That is an enormous amount of money being spent on something that, at best, produces conflicting outcomes.

Why? They simply want to satisfy the need to do something. Wellness programs that supposedly move people toward healthier lifestyles look great on reports and audits. But do the employees look great in the mirror? The largest study to date measuring the outcomes of such programs concluded that the programs do not in fact change measurable health metrics such as weight or blood pressure.[7]

Perhaps we should return to a time when insurance companies offered lower premiums for healthier people and even had their own wellness programs. I imagine if the insurance premium or amount of cost sharing decreased a substantial amount with documented weight loss and lower blood pressure, that would motivate some individuals who are straining to cover their health care costs. Conversely, if the doctor documents that their patient is continuing to smoke, use marijuana, eat a poor diet, gain weight, and poorly manage type 2 diabetes, then what if the insurance company and doctors charged more to cover such complex (costly) care? What if the responsibility was placed on the patient rather than the medical doctor for failure to meet health metrics set in place by the insurance company? Where is the tangible incentive for patients to improve themselves in this backward system of value-based care? You would think the concept of living a healthier life would motivate people but it alone does not. In fact, a onetime monetary reward will have little long-term impact. But a continuous system with positive and negative reinforcements for healthy behavior choices will directly affect health outcomes.

Is it time to use both positive and negative reinforcement in order to reduce cost and improve compliance? This is how we teach our children as they grow up, so maybe adults need to keep learning the same lessons.

If Americans would stop using tobacco, change their diets, and exercise more, 80 percent of all heart disease, stroke, and type 2 diabetes, as well as 40 percent of all cancers, may be prevented. These diseases are the biggest chunk of $150 billion per year in health care spending. We would have ample funds to develop treatments for childhood cancers, to help veterans suffering from traumatic limb amputations, to get those with mental health disorders the screening and treatment they need, to help those afflicted with traumatic brain injury, and to put the opioid crisis behind us. These goals are not beyond our grasp as a country!

The solutions are in fact quite simple. However, we lack the leadership to unify us in these goals and propel us forward to a healthier America. At one point it was our medical doctors we sought for such guidance, but as we continue down this rabbit hole of government intrusion, we are killing them off, too.

Chapter 11

PERSONAL
RESPONSIBILITY

Our society has always placed a high value on a single human life—*what can we do to cure a single person?*

Individual health is important. Equally important is making sure America remains a leader in medical innovation, with a health care system that is fiscally sustainable and a population that is not floundering in preventable illness.

Our medical system intends to deliver care, but we might as well call it "illness care." Americans are not focused on practicing healthy habits to prevent disease. We wait until we get sick, then react by getting treatment. Our insurance must pay for it, whether or not it was a preexisting condition. As a country, we need to stop this reactive pattern if we want to cut back on our outrageous costs and prevent the collapse of the entire health care system.

It is time to focus on the population group that is largely driving up prices and burdening the rest of Americans—those who are unhealthy because of the choices they make.

Punishments for Gluttons

Until about 1980, the average weight of an American adult was stable. Then we saw a sudden rise in obesity. There are many reasons why we got fat as a country, but there is one that nobody wants to talk about: the entry of women into the workforce. Don't get me wrong: I wouldn't be where I am without women's strides toward equality and independence in the twentieth century. But there are certain prices we had to pay for that independence. One of them is that fewer women, who traditionally cooked meals for their families, are doing so today. Without home cooking, we have become dependent on packaged and processed foods, notorious for higher salt and fat content.

Another reason we're overweight, and related to the first one, is that we have fast food on every corner. Takeout is a staple in most people's homes, including my own. I won't say I come home and cook dinner every night, because I don't. (In fact, my husband cooks far more often than I do.) The convenience offered by takeout, however, can feel like a lifesaver at times in a busy home.

A third reason is that we've seen a significant decline in physical activity. It comes as no surprise that our waistlines are wider than ever before. Look around you, even at the gym, and you'll see big people everywhere—60 to 75 percent of Americans are overweight or obese. This number is only increasing.

The prevalence of obesity has convinced many of us that it's acceptable. We have completely normalized being overweight with big & tall stores, "husky" jeans, plus-sized clothing, and plus-sized models. Rather than encouraging people to lower their weight to a healthy range, the market has responded by supplying the products demanded by a fat America.

Misplaced Praise?

I read an opinion piece recently by a woman who had a humiliating experience trying to board an airplane. The gate agent told her she had to buy a second seat because her girth would not fit into the economy seat she had purchased. The woman, who described herself as weighing 300 pounds, felt she was a victim of discrimination, and said so to the gate agent. She was too embarrassed by the incident to make any further commotion, so she conceded and paid for the extra seat, later detailing the account in an opinion piece. She concluded the piece by saying she is proud of her appearance and believes she deserves respect. Her piece was met with glowing praise and support for her expression of self-love.

Her choice to protest the incident to the airline was an empowering moment. Like many, I admire women with self-confidence. I love that she stood up for herself and resisted the pressure to conform to society's idea of what she should look like. At the same time, when we praise her for these qualities, we're praising a woman who is morbidly obese, and that's not okay. Yes, she is a beautiful woman. Yes, she is strong and has good self-worth. However, her obesity will lead her down a path toward illness. We want to be kind to those who aren't as healthy and fit as they should be, but are we just enabling the problem by praising such behavior?

SOUTHERN SOUL FOOD

My son is attending Ole Miss, so for his high school graduation party, I asked a caterer to bring in some southern-themed food. It was a culinary experience! We had fried chicken, gravy, mashed potatoes, macaroni and cheese, and everything else unhealthy you could imagine. For us, this was indulgence, meant for a rare celebration. In Mississippi, though, those foods are a way of life.

Given the way our country eats, it's no wonder that 50 percent of Americans have diabetes or pre-diabetes by age sixty-five.

I'm certainly not "fat-shaming" here although I don't quite understand the made-up term. This trend toward fat acceptance couldn't be more detrimental to our society. Think about it: the implication of obesity acceptance is that we're okay risking our lives with weight-related illnesses.

Are we no better than that?

Obesity and its related illnesses cost Americans approximately $150 billion every year. To put that in perspective, that's twice as much as we spend on Veterans Benefits and roughly over four times what we spend on foreign aid.[1] Individually, an obese person's medical costs are $1,429 higher than a person with normal weight. That's a lot of money for just being overweight. In other words, people are missing opportunities to work and enjoy life not because they have the flu, but because they are overweight.

Not everyone needs to be a fashion model. We don't have to strive for perfection. We just need to tip the scale slightly in our favor, literally and figuratively speaking. In fact, as little as a 5 to 10 percent reduction in weight will result in a significant improvement in medical risks for most people. Slow and steady lifestyle modifications can easily be our answer to fighting disease if we are willing to commit our country to self-restraint.

Our fatness as a nation not only translates into higher taxes, but it's undercutting our military recruiting and threatening our ability to deploy healthy troops.

The Pentagon pays roughly $1 billion a year in health care costs for obese military personnel and their families, the cost of which is nearly enough to fund the entire VA health system.[2]

Fad Diets for Fad Bodies

Thanks to our reality TV stars, we're inundated with fad weight-loss diets—low-carb this, keto that, paleo whatever. Each claim to be the best way to get rid of unwanted body fat with minimal or no sacrifice of good-tasting food. Oh, and did they mention that their diet will take no effort on your part? These diets obviously sound good to those struggling with rising poundage, but they are in fact too good to be true.

Unfortunately, even if you lose a couple of quick pounds on a fad diet, it's rarely sustainable. Most of the time, dieters return to their old habits and regain their lost weight, if not more. Can't we rid ourselves of the mentality that there's an easy fix for everything? Rome wasn't built in a day, and we can't repair our health system, inflated costs, and our individual health in a single day (or with a single legislation), either. There are no magic pills, diets, or government programs that will give the quick fix we are all seeking—we must work for it.

This is what America was built on: we work for success. If you work hard, you get rewarded. According to the Centers for Disease Control, 80 percent of Americans don't eat according to the CDC's recommended diet. We eat too many calories. Twenty-five years ago, the average American consumed about 1,850 calories per day. Now we eat over 2,000 calories, which is enough to (theoretically) add thirty-one pounds per year. Eat fewer calories, fewer processed foods, and work to keep your weight down. If you work toward healthy behaviors, you'll be rewarded with improved health, potentially increased longevity, more money in your pockets, and more time spent with your family.

Telling patients that they can make simple changes—whether it's to stop eating white bread and white potatoes or cutting out desserts and sugary drinks—to lose weight sometimes frustrates people. They believe it's more complicated than that. But most diets fail when they're impossible to follow on a daily basis. Sometimes it really is that simple to reduce weight—just by altering a few of the ways we eat.

Salt in the Wounds

Calories aside, 90 percent of Americans eat more sodium than recommended. Guess who's one of those Americans? My husband. When we got married, I never added salt to anything except hard-boiled eggs and cucumbers. Since getting married, my salt intake has increased dramatically. We get into loving arguments at times because I refuse to eat meals that he cooks with far too much salt in them.

> According to the CDC, if Americans reduced sodium intake by 1,200 mg per day, it could save up to $20 billion a year in medical costs.[3] Mind you, a regular slice of pizza averages 950 mg of sodium. Add a soda or glass of juice and you are above 1200 mg.[4]

Unfortunately, I'm the rarity. Most Americans eat as much salt as he does. Sodium can directly increase blood pressure and cause kidney damage by causing a swelling effect in the vessels, which increases the pressure. It then must be filtered through the kidneys, which results in more stress on the system. Hence, too much salt overloads the body and causes illness.

Drinking Our Weight in Sugar

Drinking sugar is as bad for us as smoking cigarettes; they both directly cause disease, and yet half of Americans drink an average of two to three sodas per day.

When Michael Bloomberg was mayor of New York City, he wanted to address rising obesity among New Yorkers. In 2012 he proposed a ban on the sale of large sodas and other sugary drinks (16 ounces or more). There was backlash, of course, and the ban was killed in the courts. To be frank, I applauded the mayor's efforts at the time. He saw the bigger picture and wanted to take action, but again, Americans rejected punitive action, especially in the form of taxation.

Reduction in sugar intake not only improves individual health but would lessen the burden on our entire system. You have every right to make poor health decisions for yourself. You can choose disease-causing behaviors as long as you are the only one affected by your decisions. These choices don't just affect the individual—they're affecting everyone.

Several American cities have imposed sugary drink taxes to reduce sugar consumption and reduce the rates of obesity and diseases like type 2 diabetes. But do you think a few extra cents is going to stop Americans from drinking what they want? Absolutely not. Yet I wonder if excluding type 2 diabetes from insurance policy coverage would be enough motivation. Under the ACA, this isn't possible, but it is this sort of negative reinforcement that we Americans apparently need to make the right decisions.

Drinking Ourselves to Death

I may not give in to salt and soda, but I would be lying if I said I didn't have a glass of wine or a cocktail a few times a week. Drinking is very much part of our social life. We have drinks after work, drinks with lunch, wine with dinner, and mimosas at brunch. The CDC says Americans spend $249 billion a year on excessive alcohol consumption.[5]

The problem is that drinking is not just a social activity. People come home from work and drink wine by themselves. Or they drink alcohol at work-related events and even on children's playdates (trust me, I know). There's a scene in the movie *Bad Moms* where the mothers go to their kids' soccer game and drink out of kids' juice cups that they've secretly filled with vodka. Outside of a funny movie, I don't think anyone would argue that drinking vodka at a child's soccer game is a good idea or beneficial to anyone's health. To relieve anxiety and boredom, it's helpful, I'm sure. Maybe we have normalized drinking alcohol, like our acceptance of obesity and America's love for soda. Are we, as in many other ways, taking personal freedom too far?

Alcohol costs us a lot of money in consequential health problems, and not just for alcoholics. It causes certain cancers, and it also contributes to obesity, car accidents, suicides, and homicides.

Between 2006 and 2015, there was a 61 percent rise in alcohol-related emergency room visits in America.[6]

More than ever, people are binge drinking and getting blackout drunk, which lands them in the hospital with alcohol poisoning. College kids come in with shock to the liver after heavy drinking, which sometimes results in long-term damage. Cirrhosis of the liver, a result of chronic alcoholism, can lead to a liver transplant, an expensive procedure that then requires long-term medication and care.

While no drinking is the best for your health, the impact of moderate drinking is much less than binge drinking. If you're not willing to give up whatever drink it is you enjoy—and my hand is raised here—we should all consider drinking a little less.

Drinking or abusing alcohol often goes along with smoking cigarettes. Both are detrimental.

The Smoking Gun

It's preposterous that people still smoke cigarettes. After all the advocacy campaigns and money that's been poured into anti-smoking efforts, people still refuse to give up this vice. Even though smokers seeking medical treatment cost our nation over $300 billion a year.[7] We also know that secondhand smoke is deadly. If you're a smoker, you're not doing anyone a favor by standing two feet away. Smoking itself kills 480,000 people per year, and secondhand smoke kills 42,000 people per year. The person who's next to you—probably your child or spouse—is still inhaling the toxins. You even have a filter on your cigarette providing some protection for yourself; they do not.

It's interesting that the people who are least able to afford cigarettes are the ones who tend to smoke. In 2014 twice as many people who had no health coverage or Medicaid smoked more than the average American. For some, they don't know better, but for the majority, it is a conscious decision to continue the addictive habit.[8]

Some people are attempting to clean up their smoking act. Vaping has picked up as the "healthy" alternative to smoking. As far as we know right now, it *is* healthier than smoking tobacco cigarettes, but cases are already piling up demonstrating lung damage and even death from vaping. Remember, just a few short decades ago, doctors used to promote smoking itself. The first ads for cigarettes had a doctor in a white coat saying, "Smoking is good for you and your lungs." Our knowledge tends to take time to catch up with our bad behaviors and even longer to change our habits. In ten years, we may be having the same conversations about vaping as we are now about cigarettes and opioids. Bottom line: don't do it. Not even socially. Inhaling anything other than the oxygen around us is undoubtedly one of the most idiotic behaviors still occurring in America, and it's costing everyone.

The Rise in Marijuana Acceptance

Speaking of understudied substances, let's talk about marijuana. Marijuana *does* have some medicinal effects. For example, it shows some benefit for people with intractable seizure disorders, or patients who have unrelenting nausea and pain, especially from cancer. However, marijuana exacerbates existing breathing problems; can lead to heart disease, psychosis, increase in fat deposition through overeating; and makes someone less likely to exercise and think clearly. There are even a few smaller studies that claim teenagers and young adults who smoke regularly have lower IQs, which parallels lower income and socioeconomic status as an adult.

For some people, marijuana may be essential. For most people, recreational marijuana use has little benefit and the potential for harm. In states where it's been legalized, at least the taxes collected on it can help pay for the illnesses it will cause. But providing additional avenues for people to get sick doesn't make sense. We have enough illness.

When the Sun Just Isn't Good Enough

Ultraviolet (UV) damage to the skin directly causes skin cancer, just as cigarette smoking causes lung cancer. Even if you don't lay out in the sun every day, simply golfing on the weekends can put you at a significantly increased risk of getting skin cancer.

Yet we somehow managed to make this concept worse—tanning beds are preposterous. I admit as an adolescent I ignorantly used a tanning bed, but as an adult, I am amazed that these still exist. Even if we took the negative effects from a tanning bed away, it is another prime example of self-indulgent behavior, causing long-term financial and health toxicity. Is the risk of skin cancer worth the reward, or have we stopped caring because, like everything else, we have normalized having skin lesions removed?

Taxation

Some have suggested taxing tanning salons, but that's the Democrats' answer for everything: *just tax it.* Like cigarettes, sugary drinks, and, now, marijuana. Taxing means the government can't trust the people to quit their own bad habits. Stop the behavior and not only will we not need the additional taxes, but we will all be better off for it.

Besides, we know a tax isn't a very good deterrent. Instead, we could require people to pay more up front for health insurance or doctor visits if they continue these behaviors that directly result in costly illness. Yet by refusing to do this, we are allowing the government to come in and force regulation on us. Perhaps we could try this: if you *choose* to use tanning beds you must sign a waiver that is uploaded into a centralized system. You not only acknowledge the risk of artificial tanning, but you also release the government and your private insurance from any costs incurred for potential future skin cancer treatment. Instead, the cost of your resultant illness will be on you. Furthermore, physicians are released from their mandate to treat your condition if you are unable to pay them. Imagine how well that scenario would be received. Something tells me this drastic measure may be more of a deterrent than a nominal tax.

If we continue to expect the government to pay for everything— and we continue to tax everything—then we're going to move away from what America was built on. We'll have a federal government that's obsessed with overregulation and a population that goes along with it.

As a physician, it's hard for me to make this distinction. On one hand, I want to tell the government to get rid of cigarettes, soda, and tanning beds, for starters. I have no idea why we have them in the first place given the fact that they have zero health benefits and loads of negative effects. On the other hand, I am proud that as Americans we have freedom of choice. Corporations also have the right to economic freedom, too. Companies can provide unhealthy substances, and Americans can choose to consume them. Similarly, private insurance companies should have the freedom not to cover people who refuse to give up their vices. Also, the rest of the American people should also have the right to not pay for other people's bad decisions. There are so many ways to prevent disease, so why aren't we doing more?

If Only There Were a Vaccine to Prevent Cancer—Oh, Wait, There Is

Earlier on, I mentioned two viruses, HPV and HBV, that, if prevented, could potentially save 60,000 people from being diagnosed with cancer every year. We have vaccines against these viruses, and most of the time, they are free. So, despite the good news, why haven't more people gotten them?

Unfortunately, despite our medical advances in vaccinations and treatments, fake news and dangerous myths about vaccines are running rampant in our communities. In 2019 measles, once considered eradicated in the United States, reappeared in emergency outbreaks throughout the country. Despite robust research dispelling the myths and falsities spread about vaccinations, we are seeing more and more parents preventing their children from being vaccinated, which will ultimately lead to disease and death. In fact, one in four people who become infected by the measles virus will need an expensive hospitalization. Our society has taken a step backward, and we are spending millions of dollars combating a virus that we had declared gone in 2000, all because of the *choice* not to vaccinate.

A little less than ten years ago, the CDC recommended eleven- and twelve-year-old girls receive the HPV vaccine. Since then, the recommendation has expanded to adults. In 2016 and 2017, only about 20 percent of adolescents got the vaccine. There are multiple reasons why: People are concerned about adverse side effects (an unfounded concern). Or they might not think their child is at risk; but children become teenagers, and any sexually active person (or even a person only going to third base) is at risk. Perhaps most likely of all: they believe Hollywood faux experts who tell them not to.

People don't even know that the HPV vaccine was made to protect our children. Human papillomavirus is a very common sexually transmitted virus, with an estimated 80 percent of sexually active people contracting it at some point in their lives. Approximately 14 million new infections occur yearly in the United States, and as I noted previously, about 79 million people, men and women, are believed to have an active HPV infection at any given time.

People should be allowed freedom of choice, but that freedom of choice doesn't always hold when our choices have the potential to cause cancer in another individual. The HPV virus not only affects the people who have it, but it can be transmitted to their sexual partners like HIV. You can try to instill safe-sex practices in your children, but when over 79 million people in the US have this virus, it will be difficult to protect them from everyone they encounter. Choosing not to protect children from HPV with a vaccine is selfish and negligent. Why say to children, "Don't smoke cigarettes because they'll cause cancer," then deny them the HPV vaccine? They are much more likely to contract HPV than to start smoking cigarettes.

It all comes down to this: you either want to protect your children or you don't.

Fixing Our Country, from the Inside Out

As a radiologist, I have the power to see people from the inside out. I see their lungs, their bones, and the tumors growing in their bodies. At times, I don't actually see the outside of the patient, but I know more about them than meets the eye. They might have a facelift, fake lips, fake hair, fake breasts, fake everything, but none of that can keep me from seeing the real person.

I don't have to wait for them to present with symptoms. I can tell them, "You're not looking good on the inside. You need to fix something, and it's not your lips." Their work on the outside might make them look younger and give them the facade of health, but everyone's insides tell the truth.

What's interesting, though, is that when I diagnose cancer, the patients always say, "I'm really healthy—how can I have cancer?" Even if she's a morbidly obese woman or smells of tobacco, I'm not going to tell her just then, "You have chosen a lifestyle that may have contributed to your disease." I'll keep my mouth shut in that moment. Not because I'm paralyzed by political correctness, but because there is no point. She has cancer, we established that fact, so it's more important to move onto illness care and treat her disease.

As Americans, we do what we want. It's one of our greatest strengths as well as one of our greatest weaknesses. We want the quick fix and none of the consequences of our bad habits. This entire health care journey is a slow and steady process, but that's the only road toward long-term success.

As a nation we are on this trek together. Partisan politics, federal legislation, and fad diets won't help us. Make the changes to be the best version of yourself to help put us on the path to a healthier America.

AFTERWORD

Life as a physician is notoriously hectic, laborious, and exhausting. Despite this workload, I find myself overwhelmingly fulfilled knowing that I help many people lead longer, healthier, and, importantly, happier lives. In some of the more challenging clinical scenarios, the physician's instincts take over to safely guide our patients through the darkest of moments. Yet I am constantly reminded of a maxim that we are taught as young physicians: We are doctors by profession, humans by emotion.

During my first rotation on the internal medicine service, I was helping to take care of a young woman who was dying from advanced pancreatic cancer, her body ravaged by the consequences of years of unbridled alcohol addiction. As if to add to this insult, she had also been admitted to the hospital with a pervasive infection of head lice. This placed her in the hospital equivalent of solitary confinement—isolation. While other medical personnel coordinated her ultimate disposition of palliative care and hospice, she sat alone, cut off from the world and ostracized by her own family.

I walked into her room one morning. After donning the yellow plastic smock, hairnet, and gloves required to enter patient's rooms according to isolation precautions, I gently pushed open her door and found her quietly staring out the window, tears pouring from her jaundiced eyes. It would be natural to assume she was in despair from having a terminal diagnosis. When Mary turned to me, I could tell there was so much more. She told me of her marriage, and how they had quickly become a family of four. She explained

how she quickly fell into a state of undiagnosed postpartum depression, self-prescribing alcohol to cope with her impaired state.
It was this solace that would ultimately take her family from her
and give her the cancer that would end her life.

Her bottle of treatment shampoo had been unceremoniously
dropped into her room, along with plastic-wrapped instructions.
In her debilitated state, she simply lacked the strength to wash
her hair full of lice. In her isolated condition, no family was coming to help her, either. She was too ashamed to tell them she was
dying, sickened by the very thing that drove them apart. So I sat
with Mary in silence, as I ran the sudsy warm water through her
thinned red hair, helping her wash away some of the pain.

Mary's situation ignited an internal struggle that to this day I
still grapple with. There is an elusive balance between compassion for an illness and the practical understanding of life choices
that may lead to that illness. Compassion is one of the staunchest
virtues of any medical mission statement, although this virtue is
impossible to instill in others and challenging to hold on to oneself
through the tests of time. Treating an infinite number of patients
with self-inflicted illness such as addictions and obesity has the
potential for eroding one's sense of compassion. How can I care for
someone if they simply do not care enough to care for themselves?
It is easy to fall into this thought process.

Compassion is the very thing that makes us human and sepa-
rates us from the rest of the animal kingdom. We treat our sick, aid
our infirm, and help those who have made mistakes. To err is to be
human, and to be American is to help our fellow man, or woman.
The mission of a physician is to engage with patients in the pursuit
of a healthy life, all the while maintaining an emotional bond with
the people who trust us with their lives.

Over a decade ago, the Italian physician Giovanni Pes and Belgian demographer Michel Poulain identified a small Sardinian region in Italy where some of the world's longest-living people resided. These "blue zones," as they would come to be known, are home to people who reach the age of 100 years at rates ten times greater than that of the US population. Researchers looking into these blue zones found that the combination of a healthier diet coupled with increased physical and social activity contributed to this longevity. The overall reduction of disease and continued sense of purpose allowed this population of centenarians to have a higher sense of life satisfaction. Sure, genetics may play a role, but according to the National Institutes of Health study on longevity, only 20 to 25 percent of one's life expectancy is predicted by genetics. A healthy lifestyle maximizing disease prevention is crucial to achieving not only a long life but a satisfying life.

We have the most sophisticated technology and extensive professional training at our fingertips, yet we habitually lack basic discipline and personal control. The essence of a doctor-patient relationship boils down to shared responsibility. Doctors can provide care, including diagnosis and treatment, as well as knowledge and compassion. The patient, however, is responsible for making the choice to adhere to medical advice, which includes embracing preventative measures and living healthier lives.

Health policy discussions are difficult because we are forcing ourselves to make emotionally trying decisions about wellness not only for ourselves but our entire society. It may be time for us as a country to embrace carrot-and-stick incentivization. To strive for equal opportunities but accept there will be varying outcomes. To agree that rewards should be given for those striving to be better.

There is no way to escape disease, and no one gets out of here alive. However, we can take control of how much of our life is spent being healthy and not suffering physically, emotionally, and financially because of unhealthy behaviors. By taking responsibility for our own actions and lessening preventable illness, we will shift resources for those that truly need it.

America may be sick, but we will survive. We have the knowledge and tools to make America healthy again. We just need to take the first step and acknowledge that much of the crisis we are in is by our own misdoing.

ACKNOWLEDGMENTS

I would not exist, literally and figuratively, if it were not for my family. The love of my parents, the support of my siblings, and the patience of my husband, all coupled with the tenacity of my children, form the foundation that made this book possible.

I am eternally grateful for the headstrong personality and adventures my father instilled in me, and the compassion and selflessness in my mother that I strive to emulate.

Early mornings and late nights have become the new normal in my household. Thank you Nicholas, Hudson, and Harrison for reminding me to stop and smell the flowers along the way in life.

For my Mommom and my Uncle Joe, who both succumbed to devastating cancers. I look forward to the day when we can refocus our efforts not only to curing cancer but preventing it altogether, so no one ever must suffer the way you did.

To my colleagues who share their experiences with me. You have inspired me to discuss the perils we are facing in today's health care paradigm. To Lauren and Suzanne, for seeing something in me I didn't know existed.

I express my gratitude to my patients, who have educated me on all facets of professional and personal responsibility; constantly reminding me why I dedicate my life to the medical profession.

APPENDIX:
AN OUTLINE FOR A
HEALTHIER LIFE

There is no magic diet, pill, or exercise that will guarantee a disease-free life. Even the most conscientious individuals who make lifestyle modifications and get recommended screenings may still get sick. However, the healthier we keep our body and mind, the better we will be at preventing disease and fighting it if it occurs. Be your best—if not for you, for those around you.

KILLER 1: CARDIOVASCULAR DISEASE

Cardiovascular disease is a term for an unhealthy heart and/or blood vessels. The Big Food industry has capitalized on our desire for certain culinary pleasures. The food and beverage industry provides us with irresistible delights in pleasingly social atmospheres. Restaurant food typically contains five to ten times the salt that you would use in preparing food at home, and hidden sugars are everywhere in the larger than necessary portions served. All of this would be fine if people were educated about what they were consuming and either avoided it altogether or were able to limit themselves to enjoy these occasions in moderation. Because of our inability to do so, cardiovascular disease and all the unhealthy components that go along with it (high blood pressure, type 2 diabetes) are epidemic in America.

The good news is, not only is much of cardiovascular disease preventable with diet, but for those who are already affected or genetically

predisposed, through monitoring and medication the unwanted consequences are largely avoidable as well. The bad news is, elevated blood
pressure and blood sugar are asymptomatic until damage is being done
and a diagnosis is inevitable.

Prevention Method One: Diet

There is no magic diet to stave off disease. Most fad diets result in immediate results with long-term failure. If you focus on three main ideas
when deciding what you consume, you are working toward long-term
success regarding your heart health.

1. Cut the Salt

A high-salt diet directly raises blood pressure by drawing more volume into our blood vessels. Even if you don't add salt to your food every
day, chances are you're still eating far too much of it. The World Health
Organization advises adults to consume less than 2 g of sodium (approx.
5 g of salt) per day for a healthy heart.

Ways to eliminate table salt from your diet:
a. If you are cooking at home, try experimenting with fresh garlic,
   lemon juice, and flavored vinegar to flavor your meals, along with
   herbs and spices such as salt-free herb blends, cumin, nutmeg, fresh
   ground pepper, tarragon, oregano, and many others.
b. If you simply are not enjoying food without adding a lot of salt, then
   switch to a lighter salt option. These are salts made up of potassium
   chloride either in addition to or rather than sodium chloride. It is
   not the same as cutting out salt altogether, but these alternatives
   have been shown in multiple international studies to effectively
   lower blood pressure. However, those with kidney problems should
   be wary of taking excess potassium, as your kidneys can't process it.
c. Focus on naturally low-sodium foods. When trying to restrict
   salt intake, remember that many foods contain it already. Read

nutrition labels and choose foods containing 140 mg or less, which is considered low-sodium.

d. Add fresh fruits, vegetables, whole grains, and legumes (dried beans, lentils, split peas) into your reduced-sodium diet.

SAPHIER SAYS: Make it a goal to incorporate naturally low-sodium foods over a couple weeks into your diet. Gradually experiment with using a lighter salt or salt-free herbs and spices in your favorite recipes rather than traditional salt. Try to decrease the frequency of eating out to one or two times per week, but if you must, ask for low-salt options. Soon you won't even miss the taste of salt at all.

2. Avoid Blood-Sugar Spikes

Fluctuations in blood sugar affect us all, whether we have a diagnosis of diabetes or not. High levels of sugar in the blood vessels cause direct damage to the lining and also increase the risk of blood clots, which may block blood flow, leading to heart attacks, strokes, and other catastrophic events. Type 2 diabetes occurs when the body has had high levels of blood sugar for a while, which leads to the body's resistance to its own insulin (the natural hormone that regulates our blood sugar). Unfortunately, people are not paying attention to their blood-sugar fluctuations until they are symptomatic (e.g., high blood pressure) and already have type 2 diabetes. With diabetes being one of the most expensive diseases in America, we should start paying attention to our blood-sugar levels long before even pre-diabetes occurs.

Ways to naturally stabilize blood sugar:

a. Increase your intake of vegetables, greens (kale, spinach), and whole-grain fiber foods. These have lower carbohydrates and therefore do not cause drastic increases in blood sugars.

b. Get enough protein by eating fish, chicken, and plant-based proteins.

c. Add some vinegar! Just 2 ounces of apple cider vinegar before bed improves fasting morning blood sugar and insulin sensitivity. If consumed prior to a meal it has been shown to reduce blood sugar following a meal by up to 34 percent. (This is not recommended in those with type 1 diabetes.)

d. Don't drink alcohol on an empty stomach because this may cause drastic fluctuations in blood sugar.

e. Avoid starchy carbohydrates such as processed white breads, potatoes, and sugary desserts to avoid spikes in blood sugar.

WARNING SIGNS OF PRE-DIABETES/TYPE 2 DIABETES

- Frequent urination (polyuria): The sugar in your blood is filtered through your kidneys. The increased sugar content draws the water with it into the kidneys, causing increased urination.

- Increased thirst (polydipsia) and dry mouth: Increased urination leaves your body dehydrated.

- Unexplained weight loss: This is typically caused by dehydration from the increased urination.

- Increased hunger, especially after a meal: When your body is no longer sensitive to insulin or not producing it, the body can't convert food consumed into energy. The lack of energy causes you to be hungry.

- Fatigue: As with increased hunger, your body is having difficulty converting food into energy, which causes tiredness.

- Headaches and blurred vision: Swelling of the optic (eye) nerve can cause vision to blur as well as headaches. Dehydration can also lead to headaches.

SAPHIER SAYS: If you are having any or a combination of these symptoms it is important to go to a medical doctor who can do a proper workup. As with cancer and other diseases, type 2 diabetes is better treated (and sometimes even cured) when diagnosed early with prompt intervention.

3. Hydrate with Water and Limit Everything Else

Water is important for your overall health and is the best source of hydration for your body.

Tips for sticking to water:

a. Add a twist of fresh lemon or lime if you need the extra flavor. Be careful of flavored and sparkling waters because some have high levels of salt and sugar in them, so check the label!

b. Cut out soft drinks, sugary smoothies, and heavily sweetened coffee drinks.

c. If you are a coffee drinker, that's good, because it has innumerable health benefits, but don't add things to it. Anything in a paper or plastic container should not be added to your coffee. In fact, slowly work up to not adding anything to your coffee. Make it a quest to find a brew you enjoy without the additives that not only alter the natural flavor of the coffee but turn what could be a healthy morning treat into a massive blood-sugar spike.

Prevention Method Two: Physical Activity

Technology and the resultant sedentary lifestyle are killing us—literally—so get moving.

Did you know evidence suggests that push-up capacity could be an easy, no-cost method to help assess cardiovascular disease risk in almost any setting? A study conducted by researchers at the Harvard T.H. Chan School of Public Health evaluated male firefighters over a ten-year period. Those who could do more than forty push-ups during a timed test at a preliminary examination were 96 percent less likely to have developed a cardiovascular problem compared to those who could do ten or less initially.

Okay, this isn't evidence-based science here, but how many uninterrupted push-ups can you do? If you are closer to forty, you are on the right track. If you are closer to ten, you have some work to do. In an effort not to be a complete hypocrite, before I sent the results of this study out on social media encouraging people to try the challenge, I decided to livestream myself from my medical office space doing uninterrupted push-ups. Forty. Phew. My arms were shaking, and I wasn't sure I would make it, but I did. Now my goal is to make sure I can always get to forty, because as we age, it will only get harder.

1. Make Exercise a Part of Your Life and Not a Chore
a. Stop using ATMs/drive-throughs.
b. Park toward the end of the parking lot.
c. Is it walkable? Skip the car and walk.
d. Take a walk around your office parking lot at least twice daily while working if you can.
e. Have a long commute? Make sure you tap your feet to keep blood flowing and your metabolism active. Do five to ten jumping jacks before and after the commute to remind your body it's alive.
f. For maximum health benefits, at least 150 minutes of moderate activity or 75 minutes of vigorous activity per week is recommended. Don't let those numbers intimidate you: 150 minutes of moderate activity can be 21 minutes per day of power walking or the 75 minutes of vigorous activity can be 11 minutes of running stairs each day. Eleven minutes a day!

SAPHIER SAYS: By including your family and friends in your exercise routine you are not only making it more enjoyable for yourself, but you are instilling healthy behaviors and habits in them. It can be done in any way—in the comfort of your home, at a gym, in a park. Consider doing it with a colleague to hold each other accountable. Make it fun. It doesn't have to be a rigid fitness routine—consider a family bike ride or hike.

Prevention Method Three: Mental Health

Stress takes a toll on your heart health and can affect your blood pressure levels at any age.

1. Reduce Stress

a. During the day it can be relaxing to take a few quiet moments for deep breathing or physical exercise. The natural endorphins and other hormones released are beneficial for mental and physical health.

b. Sleep deprivation can lead to stress, weight gain, high blood pressure, insulin resistance, type 2 diabetes, and cardiovascular disease. Sleep affects your blood pressure, too, and getting the right amount of sleep is directly linked to your heart health.

c. A regular bedtime benefits not only children but adults, too. Research shows that going to bed and waking up at the same time every day is a healthier option. A regular bedtime keeps the heart and metabolism healthy. People who go to bed at irregular times are more likely to be overweight and have high blood sugar and high blood pressure. These people are also more likely to have a heart attack or stroke than people with regular sleep patterns.

Prevention Method Four: Monitor Your Health

a. Get an annual physical exam to check for signs of disease. With more people now classified as hypertensive, doctors will need to screen more patients during their routine visits. With the lower thresholds for diagnosing high blood pressure, more patients will need to be treated with medication, receive more frequent doctor checkups and work to lower their blood pressure. As a result, doctors will need to spend more time with patients who were previously considered low risk but are now classified as hypertensive.

b. Self-monitoring promotes individual responsibility and freedom. Self-monitoring can give you a stronger sense of responsibility for your health. You may feel even more motivated to control your blood pressure with an improved diet, physical activity, and proper medication use.

c. Physical activity monitors (Fitbit, Apple Watch, etc.) and blood pressure monitors are available widely and without a prescription. Home monitoring is an easy step toward improving your health and holding yourself accountable.

d. Measuring your blood pressure frequently can result in early detection of a problem. Monitoring on a regular basis can alert you to any changes in your blood pressure earlier, which can be acted on faster.

e. Many people suffer from "white coat syndrome," in which anxiety is induced by health care environments and causes elevated blood pressure readings in patients whose blood pressure is much lower outside the doctor's office. By measuring blood pressure only at the doctor's office, these patients might be misdiagnosed. The opposite phenomenon is called "masked hypertension," where normally hypertensive patients do not exhibit high blood pressure readings under certain conditions. Monitoring your own blood pressure at home eliminates these problems, allowing for an easier and more accurate diagnosis.

f. Knowing your body's daily blood pressure fluctuations can promote lifestyle changes and decrease the necessity for medication. It may also alert you if your medication is not working and a change needs to be made. What is the point of taking an expensive medication if it isn't working? Get back in to see the doctor and show them your log of blood-pressure readings to see if they want to change your plan.

SAPHIER SAYS: Your blood pressure changes depending on where you are, what you are doing, and who you surround yourself with. It's common to experience higher blood pressure while traveling or in stressful situations. Keep an eye on your heart in different places and take extra care while traveling or under pressure.

Managing Your Disease

Not all cardiovascular disease is preventable. Our DNA plays an active role in how our body functions, and often a strong family history of heart disease and/or type 2 diabetes predisposes us to disease. It is important to know your risk of disease and make sure you are doing all you can do prevent it from occurring. This will drastically reduce the unwanted side effects from the disease if it develops.

a. Take medications as prescribed. If a diagnosis is made despite all possible diet and exercise changes, then medication may be necessary to avoid the lethal consequences of the disease.
b. Discuss with your doctor the risks and benefits of taking any medication and make sure you understand them.
c. Discuss with the pharmacist how the medication is working to keep you healthy. If you understand the mechanism, you are more inclined to take it.
d. If the drug is too expensive or not covered under your insurance:
   i.   Ask the pharmacist what the cash price is for it. Call several other pharmacy chains and compare cash prices. Did you know occasionally paying cash for your medicine is less expensive than the co-pay your insurance charges you?
   ii. Call your doctor immediately and inform them of the financial hardship regarding this medication. Often there are other drugs they can prescribe that will be covered or are less costly and will have the same effect.
   iii. If there isn't a similar medication you can take, ask if the doctor's office is able to help with a prior authorization from your insurance company. The pharmacist may also be able to help with this. You should be calling your insurance company, too.

    iv. If the doctor, insurance company, and pharmacies aren't helping, call the drug manufacturer to see if there are coupons or discounts.

SAPHIER SAYS: If you are prescribed a medication, not taking it is the worst thing you can do for yourself. There are hidden discounts everywhere, and there are people around you to help. You just need to demand it.

KILLER 2: CANCER

Prevention Method One: Diet

A healthy diet cannot guarantee cancer prevention, but it can reduce your risk of developing it.

a. Eat the colors of the rainbow—fill your plate with colorful fruits and vegetables and other plant-based foods such as whole grains and legumes.
b. Limit processed and red meats, which have both been directly linked to increased risk of various cancers.
c. Any amount of alcohol has been shown to increase the risk of some cancers, but if you choose to drink alcohol, limit your intake.
    i. Breast, colon, lung, kidney, and liver cancers are all linked to alcohol and getting them increases with the amount you drink and the length of time you have been consuming alcohol.
    ii. Take folic acid daily if you consume alcohol so your cells are not depleted of this necessary vitamin.

Prevention Method Two: Exercise

a. Obesity directly increases the risk of some cancers including breast, uterine, colon, and liver. One reason is that fat cells produce estrogen (in men and women), and an increase of estrogen can cause cancer.

b. At least thirty minutes of physical activity a day is associated with a lower cancer risk.

Prevention Method Three: Avoid Risky Behaviors

a. Avoid tobacco: All forms of tobacco use are linked directly to nearly every type of cancer. There is no safe level of tobacco use.

b. Skin cancer is one of the most common (and preventable) types of cancer. Avoid midday sun, stay out of tanning beds, wear sunglasses, use sunscreen, and wear a wide-brimmed hat when outdoors.

c. Limit sexual partners and practice safe sex with condoms. The more sexual partners you have in your lifetime the more likely you are to be infected with a sexually transmitted virus. Sexually transmitted viruses such as HPV and HIV are linked to many types of cancers such as lymphoma and sarcoma, as well as oral, throat, esophageal, penile, vaginal, anal, and cervical cancers. Birth control (oral contraceptives, IUDs) and abortion pills do not prevent sexually transmitted diseases. Only condoms have shown to decrease the risk of transmittance. The viruses can be shared through oral sex as well.

d. Do not share needles. Intravenous drug users have a higher risk of contracting certain viruses such as hepatitis B and C, which can lead to liver cancer. HIV can also be spread this way. Although cessation of IV drug use is preferable, safe needle practices are encouraged to lessen the spread of infection.

e. Vaccinate.

  i. HPV

  • The last two decades have proven that the human papilloma virus (HPV) is the direct cause of some of the worst cancers we suffer from, including many of the devastating head and neck cancers as well as cervical and anal cancers. Our research and development have provided us with a vaccination for adolescents to prevent infection and subsequent cancers from this common virus.

- HPV itself is asymptomatic. Men typically do not even know they carry the virus.
- Not everyone who contracts the virus will develop cancer, but nearly 100 percent of all cervical cancers are from HPV. So if we eliminate HPV, we may also be eliminating cervical (among other) cancers. Australia is on track to have completely eradicated cervical cancer with a national implementation of the vaccine when it was first approved. America lags because of many unfounded anti-vaccine campaigns.
- Boys and girls ages eleven and twelve are recommended to receive the vaccine. The recommendation is to obtain the vaccine during adolescence, before becoming sexually active; however, the FDA approves receiving it until age forty-five for men and women. There are thousands of varying strains of HPV, so even if you have already been infected by it, receiving the vaccine will protect you from many other strains that could lead to cancer. The earlier you receive the vaccine, the better chance of avoiding this deadly virus.

ii. Hepatitis B

- Hepatitis B drastically increases the risk of liver cancer but is far less common than the HPV infection.
- The vaccination is recommended in certain high-risk groups such as health care workers, sexually active but not monogamous adults, people with STDs, and IV drug users.

SAPHIER SAYS: For those who have switched from traditional tobacco cigarettes to e-cigarettes/vapes, you are eliminating (as far as we know) the cancer-causing effects of the harmful tobacco and various chemicals contained within it. However, the nicotine in the e-cigarettes causes blood vessel damage and increases blood sugar, both resulting in cardiovascular disease. Also, the flavoring chemical in the popular vapes is being heavily investigated for causing severe lung damage in several people, resulting in respiratory failure and death.

Prevention Method Four: Monitor Your Health

1. Annual Physical Exams

a. Family history of cancer is crucial to assess risk.

b. Consider genetic testing. If there is a strong family history of cancer, a genetic mutation may be present. Having knowledge of this mutation allows families not only to do aggressive screening for cancers but prompts discussion of risk-reducing treatments to eliminate the chance of a certain cancer altogether.

c. Physical examinations are advised to look for signs of disease.

Not all cancer is preventable. Our DNA plays an active role in how our body functions, and often a strong family history of cancer or a genetic mutation predisposes us to disease. It is important to know the risk of disease and make sure you are doing all you can to prevent it or detect it as early as possible through screening. Because many cancers can be cured if diagnosed early, screening programs have been initiated to do so, especially in the most common cancers.

2. Recognize Types of Cancers

a. Breast

    i. One in eight women will be diagnosed with breast cancer over the course of her lifetime.

    ii. Early detection through screening programs and improved treatments have decreased the number of people who die from this disease. The earlier it is detected, the easier it is to treat and provides the best possible chance of survival.

    iii. Only 15 percent of women who get breast cancer have a family history.

    iv. Just under 1 percent of all breast cancer occurs in men. African American women tend to get more aggressive breast cancers.

b. Colon

    i. One of the most curable cancers if diagnosed early. One of the deadliest if diagnosed late.

ii. Increasing numbers of young people (<40 years old) are being diagnosed. A diet rich in red meat is thought to be linked to the increase in colon cancers.

iii. Traditional direct visualization colonoscopy remains the standard of care. It is recommended that people begin testing at age 45 if there is no strong family history of disease. Other options include a new CT scan called virtual colonoscopy.

SAPHIER SAYS: A virtual colonoscopy is a great option if you are forgoing colon cancer screening because you reject the concept of a camera in your nether-regions. However, the colon cleansing you do to prepare for the traditional colonoscopy leaves you a couple pounds lighter and removes years of toxin buildup in your colon.

c. Lung
   i. The most common cancer people die from.
   ii. Most lung cancers today are not linked to cigarette smoking but to other environmental factors such as pollution and occupational exposure.
   iii. Low radiation dose CT scans are now being performed in high-risk people (smokers, former smokers, those with chronic lung disease).

d. Skin
   i. Most skin cancers in adulthood develop from the damage done in our youth.
   ii. You know your body better than anyone. If you see something new on your body, go see your primary-care doctor or dermatologist.
   iii. If you have a family history of skin cancer or are frequently exposed to the sun, consider annual skin checks by a dermatologist.

SAPHIER SAYS: If you consistently have nail polish on your fingers and toes, make sure to take a quick look during polish changes because small melanomas can develop under your nail bed. They look like a bruise (as if you slammed your finger in the door) but can be deadly. Also, when you are at the gynecologist, ask your doctor to check the area because melanoma can also develop around the vagina.

e. Cervical
  i. Having fewer sexual partners reduces the risk. Use condoms to decrease the chance of contracting HPV.
  ii. Get Pap smears on the recommended schedule to screen for HPV infection and cellular changes from the virus.
  iii. Get the HPV vaccine.

Managing the Disease

It shouldn't take a cancer diagnosis to prompt a healthier lifestyle. However, survivability in cancer patients is linked to mental health, healthier diet, and regular exercise, even after the diagnosis.

a. Strengthen your support system.
  i. Consider getting a dog. Studies have shown that patients with dogs as pets have overall improved emotional health.
  ii. Everyone is affected by a cancer diagnosis. It is crucial that caregivers, spouses, children, and other loved ones feel a part of the process. Not only does it help them to cope, but it helps the patient as a support.
  iii. Consult a dietician/nutritionist. Often at the same medical facility where cancer is being treated, there is a nutritionist on staff to provide guidance and health tips. If not available, reputable organizations provide information on their websites.

iv. Find exercise that works for you.
- Yoga can be specifically tailored for those with cancer. If you can't find this kind of yoga class, consider going to a session dedicated to pregnant women, as they often go at a slower pace and you can do what you feel comfortable with.
- Walk outside. Not only is walking good for your health, but being in nature (if you live in a city, go to the park) has repeatedly been shown to help with mental health and overall wellness.

Mental Health

Major mental illnesses such as schizophrenia and bipolar disorder usually develop gradually. Often, family and friends recognize subtle changes in a person's thinking or behavior before the full-blown illness appears.

Recognizing early warning signs and performing early intervention can help reduce the severity of an illness and may even delay or prevent a major mental illness altogether. If several of the following are occurring, it may be necessary to get a mental health evaluation:

- Sleep or appetite changes
- Mood changes
- Social withdrawal
- Decreased academic and/or social functioning
- Illogical thinking or confusion
- Increased sensitivity
- Nervousness
- Uncharacteristic behavior

One or two of these symptoms alone can't predict a mental illness but may indicate a need for further evaluation. People with suicidal thoughts or intent, or thoughts of harming others, need immediate attention.

SAPHIER SAYS: There are simple things we can all do to make sure that we're doing our best mentally and emotionally, like exercising, getting enough sleep, and spending enough time alone to reflect on our self. Schedule some leisure time. Work on your breathing. Take a vacation from electronic devices, even if it's just for twenty minutes in the evening. And if you are ever prescribed medication, please take it. If you disagree with the diagnosis or medication recommendation, get a second opinion but don't write off what your health care professionals are recommending. Do the simple things to clean up your mental and emotional well-being.

OPIOID CRISIS/CHRONIC PAIN

Anyone who takes opioids is at risk for becoming addicted. Opioids trigger the release of endorphins, the reward centers in the brain, which is what makes them so addictive.

a. Factors that put someone at an increased risk of becoming addicted:
   i. Family or personal history of substance abuse
   ii. Unemployment
   iii. Poverty
   iv. History of depression or anxiety
   v. Heavy tobacco use
b. How to avoid becoming addicted:
   i. Avoid long-term use. Taking opioids for more than three days significantly increases the risk of becoming addicted.
   ii. If you are undergoing surgery or suffer from chronic pain and will be prescribed opioids, discuss alternative pain control options with the doctor.
   iii. If you have been prescribed opioids and run out of the medication while still in need of pain control, ask for an alternative pain control option rather than refilling the opioid prescription.

c. What can we do about those already addicted?

  i. Seeking professional addiction counseling is essential to overcome an opioid addiction. Call your insurance company to ask about treatment centers in the network. If they do not cover addiction services, the Department of Health and Human Services in your state will find you help and assist in the cost.

- Outpatient programs
- Residential programs (more intensive and often more effective than outpatient programs)
- Medically monitored detoxification: The detoxification process can be severe and have dangerous health implications. If you do it under professional guidance, doctors can help alleviate the unpleasant effects, which will not only keep you safe but decrease the chance of relapse.

SAPHIER SAYS: When it comes to the opioid crisis, we are all drinking from the same well and we are also all contributing to polluting the water. Whether you are the prescribing doctor, the supplying pharmaceutical company, the person addicted, or the employer of the addicted, we must all stand up to support those who need treatment and do our part to stop future addictions.

DOCTOR BURNOUT

SAPHIER SAYS: Physicians have to take control of their profession. We are letting ourselves be held hostage by the concept that everyone is replaceable, that if we say no to an administrator's directive, someone else will do our job for less money. It is time to band together through organizations free from political connections. As a profession, we should consider teaming up with the FAIR Health initiative to set regional standards regarding compensation and quality metrics rather than allowing third parties like large insurance companies and the government to dictate what our time is worth. We have allowed ourselves to become a fragmented profession that caters to large third-party payers rather than our patients. If we work together, we can be a more powerful force to combat these larger entities.

Think outside of the box in terms of your practice. Is it possible to implement direct primary care (DPC) for your patients without utilizing third-party insurers? For those in a situation like mine, a specialist at a large cancer treatment and research center, DPC is not practical. But for other physicians, it may offer a better way.

Our time, health, and happiness are invaluable, so we need to learn to say no more often. We need to stop putting ourselves in situations where we feel expendable and taken advantage of. For the nonphysicians reading this, please remember that your doctor is a human being who has dedicated his or her life to help people like you. The vast majority of your experience in the medical system is out of our control, but please do voice your concerns to us so we understand you better and can, in turn, help you.

RESOURCES

HEART HEALTH:

http://www.nsc.org/Connect/NSCNewsReleases/Lists/Posts/Post
.aspx?ID=263

https://www.healthsystemtracker.org/chart-collection/mortality-rates
-u-s-compare-countries/#item-u-s-highest-rate-deaths-amenable
-health-care-among-comparable-oecd-countries

MENTAL HEALTH:

https://www.nami.org/Learn-More/Mental-Health-By-the-Numbers

https://www.ncbi.nlm.nih.gov/pmc/articles/PMC1563985/

https://www.nasmhpd.org/docs/publications/MDCdocs/Mortality%20
and%20Morbidity%20Final%20Report%208.18.08.pdf

https://jamanetwork.com/journals/jamapsychiatry/
fullarticle/208671

https://adaa.org/about-adaa/press-room/facts-statistics#

TOBACCO USE:

https://www.ncbi.nlm.nih.gov/pmc/articles/PMC4862676/

NOTES

INTRODUCTION
1. Cynthia Koons and Robert Langreth, "How Marketing Turned the EpiPen into a Billion-Dollar Business," Bloomberg, September 23, 2015, https://www.bloomberg .com/news/articles/2015-09-23/how-marketing-turned-the-epipen-into-a-billion -dollar-business.
2. "Kenneth C. Frazier, Executive Compensation," Salary. https://www1.salary.com /Kenneth-C-Frazier-Salary-Bonus-Stock-Options-for-MERCK-and-CO.html.

CHAPTER 1: THE AMERICAN HEALTH CRISIS
1. "Remarks by the President to a Joint Session of Congress on Health Care," Obama White House archives, September 9, 2009, https://obamawhitehouse.archives.gov /the-press-office/remarks-president-a-joint-session-congress-health-care.
2. "Historical," Centers for Medicare & Medicaid Services, December 11, 2018, https://www.cms.gov/Research-Statistics-Data-and-Systems/Statistics-Trends -and-Reports/NationalHealthExpendData/NationalHealthAccountsHistorical .html; John Tozzi, "Employees' Share of Health Costs Continues Rising Faster Than Wages," *Insurance Journal*, October 8, 2018, https://www.insurancejournal.com /news/national/2018/10/08/503575.htm.
3. Austin Frakt, "Medical Mystery: Something Happened to U.S. Health Spending After 1980," *New York Times*, May 14, 2018, https://www.nytimes.com/2018/05/14 /upshot/medical-mystery-health-spending-1980.html?module=inline.
4. Sarah Kliff, "I Read 1,182 Emergency Room Bills This Year. Here's What I Learned," *Vox*, December 18, 2018, https://www.vox.com/health-care/2018/12/18/18134825 /emergency-room-bills-health-care-costs-america.
5. Cheryl D. Fryar, Jeffery P. Hughes, Kirsten A. Herrick, and Namanjeet Ahluwalia, "Fast Food Consumption Among Adults in the United States, 2013–2016," Centers for Disease Control and Prevention, NCHS Data Brief No. 322, October 2018, https://www.cdc.gov/nchs/products/databriefs/db322.htm.
6. Centers for Disease Control and Prevention, "Only 1 in 10 Adults Get Enough Fruits or Vegetables," press release, November 16, 2017, https://www.cdc.gov/media /releases/2017/p1116-fruit-vegetable-consumption.html.
7. American Society of Plastic Surgeons, "2018 National Plastic Surgery Statistics," 2019, https://www.plasticsurgery.org/documents/News/Statistics/2018/plastic -surgery-statistics-report-2018.pdf.
8. Alok A. Khorana, Katherine Tullio, Paul Elson, et al., "Time to Initial Cancer Treatment in the United States and Association with Survival Over Time: An Observational Study," *PLoS ONE* 14, no. 3 (2019), https://doi.org/10.1371 /journal.pone.0213209.

9.   Cancer Research UK, "Cancer Diagnosis and Treatment Statistics," August 20, 2015, https://www.cancerresearchuk.org/health-professional/cancer-statistics /diagnosis-and-treatment#heading-One.

CHAPTER 2: WHY IS HEALTH CARE SO EXPENSIVE?

1.   Health Care Cost Institute, "2017 Health Care Cost and Utilization Report," February 11, 2019, https://www.healthcostinstitute.org/research/annual-reports /entry/2017-health-care-cost-and-utilization-report.
2.   Pan American Health Organization, "Health Status of the Population: Noncommunicable Disease Prevention and Control," https://www.paho.org/salud-en-las-americas -2017/?p=1391.
3.   Laura Donnelly, "NHS Provokes Fury with Indefinite Surgery Ban for Smokers and Obese," *Telegraph*, October 17, 2017, https://www.telegraph.co.uk/news/2017 /10/17/nhs-provokes-fury-indefinite-surgery-ban-smokers-obese/.
4.   "Prevalence of Childhood Obesity in the United States," Centers for Disease Control and Prevention, June 24, 2019, https://www.cdc.gov/obesity/data /childhood.html.
5.   Partnership to Fight Chronic Disease, "Fact: Healthy Behavior and Better Treatment Critical to Lowering Health Care Costs," press release, April 19, 2016, https:// www.fightchronicdisease.org/latest-news/fact-healthy-behavior-and-better -treatment-critical-lowering-health-care-costs.

CHAPTER 3: AMERICA, YOU'RE BREAKING OUR HEART

1.   Howard G. Bruenn, "Clinical Notes on the Illness and Death of President Franklin D. Roosevelt," *Annals of Internal Medicine* 72, no. 4 (1970): 579–91; William B. Kannel, "Contribution of the Framingham Study to Preventive Cardiology," *Journal of the American College of Cardiology* 15, no. 1 (1990): 206–11.
2.   AEF: The ANA Educational Foundation, "Seat Belt Education (1985–Present)," https://aef.com/classroom-resources/social-responsibility/ad-council-campaigns -made-difference/seat-belt-education/.
3.   Centers for Disease Control and Prevention, "Heart Disease and Stroke Deaths Hitting Middle Age Adults in Large Numbers," CDC Newsroom, September 6, 2018, https://www.cdc.gov/media/releases/2018/p0906-Heart-disease-stroke -deaths.html.
4.   American Heart Association, "CDC Prevention Programs," May 18, 2018, https:// www.heart.org/en/get-involved/advocate/federal-priorities/cdc-prevention- programs.
5.   Melonie Heron, "Deaths: Leading Causes for 2014," *National Vital Statistics Report* 65, no. 5 (June 30, 2016), https://www.cdc.gov/nchs/data/nvsr/nvsr65 /nvsr65_05.pdf.
6.   Cleveland Clinic, "Study: One in Five Deaths Linked to Poor Diet," April 3, 2019, https://newsroom.clevelandclinic.org/2019/04/03/study-one-in-five-deaths -linked-to-poor-diet/.
7.   A BMI calculator is available at https://www.cdc.gov/healthyweight/assessing /bmi/adult_bmi/english_bmi_calculator/bmi_calculator.html.

8. Centers for Disease Control and Prevention, "Heart Disease Risk Factors," 2012, https://www.cdc.gov/heartdisease/risk_factors.htm.
9. Centers for Disease Control and Prevention, "Current Cigarette Smoking among Adults in the United States," 2017, https://www.cdc.gov/tobacco/data_statistics /fact_sheets/adult_data/cig_smoking/index.htm.
10. Centers for Disease Control and Prevention, "Economic Trends in Tobacco," 2017, https://www.cdc.gov/tobacco/data_statistics/fact_sheets/economics /econ_facts/index.htm#anchor_1548357936093.
11. Andrea Neiman, Todd Ruppar, Michael Ho, et al., "CDC Grand Rounds: Improving Medication Adherence for Chronic Disease Management— Innovations and Opportunities," *Morbidity and Mortality Weekly Report* 66, no. 45 (2017), DOI: http://dx.doi.org/10.15585/mmwr.mm6645a2.
12. Emelia J. Benjamin, Paul Muntner, Alvaro Alonso, et al., "Heart Disease and Stroke Statistics—2019 Update: A Report from the American Heart Association," *Circulation* 139, no. 10 (2019), https://doi.org/10.1161/CIR.0000000000000659; Marie T. Brown and Jennifer K. Bussell, "Medication Adherence: WHO Cares?" *Mayo Clinic Proceedings* 86, no. 4 (2011): 304–14, doi:10.4065/mcp.2010.0575.
13. Lisa Boylan, "The Cost of Medication Non-Adherence," National Association of Chain Drug Stores, April 20, 2017, https://www.nacds.org/news/the-cost-of -medication-non-adherence/.

CHAPTER 4: THE BIG C: CANCER

1. National Cancer Institute, "Cancer Stat Facts: Cancer of Any Site," https://seer .cancer.gov/statfacts/html/all.html.
2. Melonie Heron and Robert N. Anderson, "Changes in the Leading Cause of Death: Recent Patterns in Heart Disease and Cancer Mortality," Centers for Disease Control and Prevention, NCHS Data Brief No. 254, August 2016, https://www .cdc.gov/nchs/products/databriefs/db254.htm.
3. Centers for Disease Control and Prevention, "United States Cancer Statistics," May 28, 2019, https://www.cdc.gov/cancer/uscs/technical_notes/index.htm? CDC_AA_refVal=https%3A%2F%2Fwww.cdc.gov%2Fcancer%2Fnpcr%2 Fuscs%2Ftechnical_notes%2Findex.htm; American Cancer Society, "Cancer Facts & Figures 2019," 2019, https://www.cancer.org/content/dam/cancer-org /research/cancer-facts-and-statistics/annual-cancer-facts-and-figures/2019 /cancer-facts-and-figures-2019.pdf.
4. American Cancer Society, "Lifetime Risk of Developing or Dying from Cancer," January 4, 2018, https://www.cancer.org/cancer/cancer-basics/lifetime -probability-of-developing-or-dying-from-cancer.html.
5. National Cancer Institute, Office of Cancer Survivorship, "Statistics," November 8, 2019, https://cancercontrol.cancer.gov/ocs/statistics/index.html stats.
6. American Cancer Society, "Cancer Facts & Figures 2019," 1.
7. National Cancer Institute, "Cancer Prevalence and Cost of Care Projections," 2011, https://costprojections.cancer.gov/.
8. World Health Organization, "Early Cancer Diagnosis Saves Lives, Cuts Treatment Costs," February 3, 2017, https://www.who.int/news-room/detail/03-02-2017 -early-cancer-diagnosis-saves-lives-cuts-treatment-costs.

9. Helen Blumen, Kathryn Fitch, and Vincent Polkus, "Comparison of Treatment Costs for Breast Cancer, by Tumor Stage and Type of Service," *American Health and Drug Benefits* 9, no. 1 (2016): 23–32.

10. Joseph A. DiMasi, Henry G. Grabowski, and Ronald W. Hansen, "Innovation in the Pharmaceutical Industry: New Estimates of R&D Costs," *Journal of Health Economics* 47 (May 2016): 20–33, https://doi.org/10.1016/j.jhealeco.2016.01.012.

11. American Cancer Society, "Cancer Facts & Figures 2019,"1.

12. American Cancer Society, "Cancer Facts & Figures 2019," 1, 44.

13. Centers for Disease Control and Prevention, "Only 1 in 10 Adults Get Enough Fruits or Vegetables," press release, November 16, 2017, https://www.cdc.gov /media/releases/2017/p1116-fruit-vegetable-consumption.html.

14. Eurídice Martínez Steele, Larissa Galastri Baraldi, Maria Laura da Costa Louzada, et al., "Ultra-Processed Foods and Added Sugars in the US Diet: Evidence from a Nationally Representative Cross-Sectional Study," *BMJ Open* 6, no. 3 (2016), https://bmjopen.bmj.com/content/6/3/e009892.

15. Daniel Esau, "Viral Causes of Lymphoma: The History of Epstein-Barr Virus and Human T-Lymphotropic Virus 1,"*Virology* 8 (September 2017), https:// www.ncbi.nlm.nih.gov/pmc/articles/PMC5621661/; Martyn K. White, Joseph S. Pagano, and Kamel Khalili, "Viruses and Human Cancers: A Long Road of Discovery of Molecular Paradigms," *Clinical Microbiology Reviews* 27, no. 3 (2014): 463–81, https://www.ncbi.nlm.nih.gov/pmc/articles/PMC4135891/.

16. Eun-Kyoung Yim and Jong-Sup Park, "The Role of HPV E6 and E7 Oncoproteins in HPV-Associated Cervical Carcinogenesis," *Cancer Research and Treatment* 37, no. 6 (2005), https://www.ncbi.nlm.nih.gov/pmc/articles/PMC2785934/; Centers for Disease Control and Prevention, "Human Papillomavirus: Genital HPV Infection," fact sheet, August 20, 2019, https://www.cdc.gov/std/hpv/stdfact-hpv.htm.

17. Centers for Disease Control and Prevention, "New Study Shows HPV Vaccine Helping Lower HPV Infection Rates in Teen Girls," press release, June 19, 2013, https://www.cdc.gov/media/releases/2013/p0619-hpv-vaccinations.html; Peter Moore, "The High Cost of Cancer Treatment," *AARP The Magazine*, June 1, 2018, https://www.aarp.org/money/credit-loans-debt/info-2018/the-high-cost-of -cancer-treatment.html.

18. Centers for Disease Control and Prevention, "Hepatitis B: Are You at Risk?" June 2010, https://www.cdc.gov/hepatitis/hbv/pdfs/hepbatrisk.pdf; Sarah Schillie, Tanja Walker, Steven Veselsky, et al., "Outcomes of Infants Born to Women Infected with Hepatitis B," *Pediatrics* 135, no. 5 (2015), https://pediatrics. aappublications.org/content/135/5/e1141.

19. "Breast Cancer: Statistics," Cancer.Net, July 2019, https://www.cancer.net/ cancer-types/breast-cancer/statistics; "Lung Cancer Fact Sheet," American Lung Association, September 25, 2019, https://www.lung.org/lung-health-and-diseases /lung-disease-lookup/lung-cancer/resource-library/lung-cancer-fact-sheet.html; "Colorectal Cancer: Statistics," Cancer.Net, November 2018, https://www .cancer.net/cancer-types/colorectal-cancer/statistics.

20. Liz Highleyman, "Many Americans Missing Out on Cancer Screenings," *Cancer Health*, September 3, 2018, https://www.cancerhealth.com/article/americans -missing-cancer-screenings.

CHAPTER 5: INTO THE DEEP

1. National Institute of Mental Health, "Mental Illness," February 2019, https://www.nimh.nih.gov/health/statistics/mental-illness.shtml.
2. National Alliance on Mental Illness, "Mental Health by the Numbers," September 2019, https://www.nami.org/learn-more/mental-health-by-the-numbers.
3. National Alliance on Mental Illness, "Mental Health by the Numbers"; NAMI, "Mental Health Facts in America," https://www.nami.org/nami/media/nami-media/infographics/generalmhfacts.pdf.
4. Thomas R. Insel, "Assessing the Economic Costs of Serious Mental Illness," *American Journal of Psychiatry* 165, no. 6 (2008): 663–65, doi: 10.1176/appi.ajp.2008.08030366.
5. National Alliance on Mental Illness, "Veterans & Active Duty," https://www.nami.org/find-support/veterans-and-active-duty.
6. National Coalition for Homeless Veterans, "Background & Statistics," http://nchv.org/index.php/news/media/background_and_statistics.
7. US Department of Veterans Affairs, "VA National Veteran Suicide Data Report 2005–2016," September 2018, https://www.mentalhealth.va.gov/docs/data-sheets/OMHSP_National_Suicide_Data_Report_2005–2016_508.pdf.
8. National Alliance on Mental Illness, "Tobacco and Smoking," https://www.nami.org/learn-more/mental-health-public-policy/tobacco-and-smoking.
9. National Alliance on Mental Illness, "Juvenile Justice," https://www.nami.org/Learn-More/Mental-Health-Public-Policy/Juvenile-Justice.
10. Jean M. Twenge, "Are Mental Health Issues on the Rise?" *Psychology Today*, October 12, 2015, https://www.psychologytoday.com/us/blog/our-changing-culture/201510/are-mental-health-issues-the-rise.
11. Jessica Wright, "The Real Reasons Autism Rates Are Up in the U.S.," *Scientific American*, March 3, 2017, https://www.scientificamerican.com/article/the-real-reasons-autism-rates-are-up-in-the-u-s/.
12. American College Health Association–National College Health Assessment, "Undergraduate Student Reference Group," Fall 2018, https://www.acha.org/documents/ncha/NCHA-II_Fall_2018_Undergraduate_Reference_Group_Data_Report.pdf.
13. Jean M. Twenge, Thomas E. Joiner, Megan L. Rogers, et al., "Increases in Depressive Symptoms, Suicide-Related Outcomes, and Suicide Rates Among U.S. Adolescents After 2010 and Links to Increased New Media Screen Time," *Clinical Psychological Science* 6, no. 1 (2018): 3–17, https://doi.org/10.1177/2167702617723376.
14. Erik Peper and Richard Harvey, "Digital Addiction: Increased Loneliness, Anxiety, and Depression," *NeuroRegulation* 5, no. 1 (2018), https://www.neuroregulation.org/article/view/18189.
15. Centers for Disease Control and Prevention, National Center for Health Statistics, "Adolescent Health," 2017, https://www.cdc.gov/nchs/fastats/adolescent-health.htm.

CHAPTER 6: THE OPIOID CRISIS

1. National Institute on Drug Abuse, "Opioid Overdose Crisis," January 2019, https://www.drugabuse.gov/drugs-abuse/opioids/opioid-overdose-crisis.
2. American Psychiatric Association, "Nearly One in Three People Know Someone Addicted to Opioids; More than Half of Millennials believe It Is Easy to Get Illegal Opioids," May 7, 2018, https://www.psychiatry.org/newsroom/news -releases/nearly-one-in-three-people-know-someone-addicted-to-opioids-more -than-half-of-millennials-believe-it-is-easy-to-get-illegal-opioids.
3. National Institute on Drug Abuse, "Misuse of Prescription Drugs," December 13, 2018, https://www.drugabuse.gov/publications/research-reports/misuse -prescription-drugs.
4. S. E. Lankenau, M. Teti, K. Silva, J. Jackson Bloom, A. Harocopos, and M. Treese, "Initiation into Prescription Opioid Misuse Amongst Young Injection Drug Users," *Int J Drug Policy* 23 no.1 (2012): 37–44; National Institute on Drug Abuse, "Prescription Opioids and Heroin," January 17, 2018, https://www.drugabuse .gov/publications/research-reports/prescription-opioids-heroin.
5. American Society of Addiction Medicine, "Opioid Addiction: 2016 Facts & Figures," https://www.asam.org/docs/default-source/advocacy/opioid-addiction -disease-facts-figures.pdf.
6. US Department of Health and Human Services, "Trump Administration Awards Grants to States to Combat Opioid Crisis," press release, April 19, 2017, https:// www.hhs.gov/about/news/2017/04/19/trump-administration-awards-grants -states-combat-opioid-crisis.html; US Department of Justice, "Attorney General Sessions Announces Opioid Fraud and Abuse Detection Unit," press release, August 2, 2017, https://www.justice.gov/opa/pr/attorney-general-sessions -announces-opioid-fraud-and-abuse-detection-unit.
7. See, e.g., Gary A. Zarkin, Alexander J. Cowell, Katherine A. Hicks, et al. "Lifetime Benefits and Costs of Diverting Substance-Abusing Offenders from State Prison," *Crime and Delinquency* 61, no. 6 (2015): 829–50.
8. James Dahlhamer et al., "Prevalence of Chronic Pain and High-Impact Chronic Pain Among Adults," *Morbidity and Mortality Weekly Report* 67, no. 36 (September 14, 2018): 1001–6.

CHAPTER 7: THE AFFORDABLE CARE ACT

1. "Average General Annual Health Plan Deductibles for Single Coverage, 2006– 2017," Kaiser/HRET Survey of Employer-Sponsored Health Benefits, https:// www.kff.org/report-section/ehbs-2017-section-7-employee-cost-sharing /attachment/figure%207_10-11/.
2. Gary Claxton, Larry Levitt, Matthew Rae, and Bradley Sawyer, "Increases in Cost-Sharing Payments Continue to Outpace Wage Growth," Peterson-Kaiser Health System Tracker, June 15, 2018, https://www.healthsystemtracker.org /brief/increases-in-cost-sharing-payments-have-far-outpaced-wage-growth/.
3. National Conference of State Legislatures, "Health Insurance: Premiums and Increases," December 4, 2018, http://www.ncsl.org/research/health/health -insurance-premiums.aspx.

4. Susan L. Hayes, Sara R. Collins, and David C. Radley, "How Much U.S. Households with Employer Insurance Spend on Premiums and Out-of-Pocket Costs: A State-by-State Look, Commonwealth Fund, May 2019.

5. United HealthCare, "IRS Sets New 2020 Limits for Group Plans and HDHP /HSA Plans," June 12, 2019, https://www.uhc.com/employer/news/midsized -business/irs-sets-new-2020-limits-for-group-plans-and-hdhp-hsa-plans; Michelle Andrews, "Federal Rule Allows Higher Out-of-Pocket Spending for One Year," *Kaiser Health News*, June 11, 2013, https://khn.org/news/061113 -michelle-andrews-out-of-pocket-costs/.

6. Michael Brady, "IRS Says Reinstating ACA Insurance Tax Would Cost Insurers $15.5B in 2020," *Modern Healthcare*, September 4, 2019, https://www.modern healthcare.com/insurance/irs-says-reinstating-aca-insurance-tax-would-cost -insurers-155b-2020.

7. Department of Health and Human Services, "Patient Protection and Affordable Care Act; HHS Notice of Benefit and Payment Parameters for 2020," April 25, 2019, https://s3.amazonaws.com/public-inspection.federalregister.gov/2019 –08017.pdf.

8. Kaiser Family Foundation, "Counties at Risk of Having No Insurer on the Marketplace (Exchange) in 2018," August 18, 2017, https://www.kff.org/interactive /counties-at-risk-of-having-no-insurer-on-the-marketplace-exchange-in-2018/.

9. Rachel Fehr, Cynthia Cox, and Larry Levitt, "Insurer Participation on ACA Marketplaces, 2014–2019," Kaiser Family Foundation, November 14, 2019, https://www.kff.org/health-reform/issue-brief/insurer-participation-on-aca -marketplaces-2014-2019/.

10. Kelsey Waddill, "ACA Premiums Will Fall 4% and 20 Payers Join Marketplace in 2020," *Health Payer Intelligence*, October 25, 2019, https:// healthpayerintelligence.com/news/aca-premiums-will-fall-4-and-20-payers -join-marketplace-in-2020.

11. Michael F. Cannon, "Is Obamacare Harming Quality?" *Health Affairs*, January 4, 2018, https://www.healthaffairs.org/do/10.1377/hblog20180103.261091/full/.

12. Kevin Williamson, "The Facts about Medicaid Fraud," *National Review*, September 11, 2016, https://www.nationalreview.com/2016/09/medicaid-fraud -staggering-cost-140-billion/.

13. Jackson Healthcare, "Physician Compensation Eight Percent of Healthcare Costs," May 26, 2011, https://jacksonhealthcare.com/media-room/news/md-salaries -as-percent-of-costs.

14. Bradley Sawyer and Cynthia Cox, "How Does Health Spending in the U.S. Compare to Other Countries?" Peterson-Kaiser Health System Tracker, December 7, 2018, https://www.healthsystemtracker.org/chart-collection /health-spending-u-s-compare-countries/#item-average-wealthy-countries -spend-half-much-per-person-health-u-s-spendshttps://www.healthsystemtracker .org/chart-collection/health-spending-u-s-compare-countries/#item-average -wealthy-countries-spend-half-much-per-person-health-u-s-spends.

15. Benjamin J. Brown, "The Deceptive Income of Physicians," *MD Magazine*, February 10, 2011, https://www.mdmag.com/journals/md-magazine/2010 /vol1-issue3/the_deceptive_income_of_physicians.

16. Teddy Nykiel, "Average Medical School Debt in 2018," NerdWallet, December 4, 2018, https://www.nerdwallet.com/blog/loans/student-loans/average-medical -school-debt/.

17. Advisory Board, "The Strikingly High Administrative Costs of US Health Care, in 3 Charts," July 23, 2018, https://www.advisory.com/daily-briefing/2018/07/23 /administrative-costs.

18. Joshua D. Gottlieb, Adam Hale Shapiro, and Abe Dunn, "The Complexity of Billing and Paying for Physician Care," *Health Affairs* 37, no. 4 (April 2018), https://doi.org/10.1377/hlthaff.2017.1325.

19. Phillip Tseng, Robert S. Kaplan, Barak D. Richman, et al., "Administrative Costs Associated with Physician Billing and Insurance-Related Activities at an Academic Health Care System," *JAMA* 319, no. 7 (2018): 691–97, doi:10.1001/jama.2017.19148.

20. James G. Kahn, "Excess Administrative Costs," in Pierre L. Young, Robert S. Saunders, and LeighAnne Olsen, eds., *The Healthcare Imperative: Lowering Costs and Improving Outcomes: Workshop Series Summary* (Washington: National Academies Press, 2010), https://www.ncbi.nlm.nih.gov/books/NBK53942/.

21. Emily Gee and Topher Spiro, "Excess Administrative Costs Burden the U.S. Health Care System," Center for American Progress, April 8, 2019, https://www .americanprogress.org/issues/healthcare/reports/2019/04/08/468302/excess -administrative-costs-burden-u-s-health-care-system/.

22. James G. Kahn, "Excess Administrative Costs."

23. Robert Langreth, "Drug Prices," *Bloomberg*, February 5, 2019, https://www .bloomberg.com/quicktake/drug-prices.

24. Ibid.

25. Kaiser Family Foundation, "Considerable Spending Variation Exists Among the Elderly, Who See the Highest Proportion of Health Spending Overall," https:// www.healthsystemtracker.org/chart-collection/health-expenditures-vary -across-population/#item-considerable-spending-variation-exists-among-the -elderly-who-see-the-highest-proportion-of-health-spending-overall_2016.

26. Julie Beck, "Less Than 3 Percent of Americans Live a 'Healthy Lifestyle,'" *The Atlantic*, March 23, 2016, https://www.theatlantic.com/health/archive/2016/03 /less-than-3-percent-of-americans-live-a-healthy-lifestyle/475065.

27. E. J. Benjamin, S. S. Virani, C. W. Callaway, et al., "Heart Disease and Stroke Statistics 2018 At-a-Glance," American Heart Association/American Stroke Association, January 31, 2018, https://healthmetrics.heart.org/wp-content /uploads/2018/02/At-A-Glance-Heart-Disease-and-Stroke-Statistics-2018.pdf.

28. American Heart Association, "CDC Prevention Programs," May 18, 2018, https:// www.heart.org/en/get-involved/advocate/federal-priorities/cdc-prevention -programs.

29. National Cancer Institute, "Cancer Prevalence and Cost of Care Projections," 2011, https://costprojections.cancer.gov/.

CHAPTER 8: THE MEDICAL DOCTOR

1. Lee Hieb, "Why the AMA Endorses Obamacare—But Your Doctor Does Not," *The Blaze*, November 6, 2012, https://www.theblaze.com/contributions/why -the-ama-endorses-obamacare-but-your-doctor-does-not.

2. Roger Collier, "American Medical Association Membership Woes Continue," *CMAJ* 183, no. 11 (2011): E713–E714, doi: 10.1503/cmaj.109–3943.

3. Peterson-Kaiser Health System Tracker, "Physicians Per Capita," https://www .healthsystemtracker.org/indicator/quality/physicians-per-capita/.

4. Blake Farmer, "When Doctors Struggle with Suicide, Their Profession Often Fails Them," NPR, July 31, 2018, https://www.npr.org/sections/health-shots /2018/07/31/634217947/to-prevent-doctor-suicides-medical-industry-rethinks-how-doctors-work.

5. "Health: Lobbying, 2019," Center for Responsive Politics, https://www .opensecrets.org/industries/lobbying.php?cycle=2020&ind=H.

6. Spencer Sutherland, "Survey Finds Nearly Half of Nurses Considering Leaving the Profession," RNnetwork, February 28, 2017, https://rnnetwork.com/blog /rnnetwork-nurse-survey/.

CHAPTER 9: WITH FREEDOM COMES RESPONSIBILITY

1. Centers for Disease Control and Prevention, "Up to 40 Percent of Annual Deaths from Each of Five Leading US Causes Are Preventable," May 1, 2014. https:// www.cdc.gov/media/releases/2014/p0501-preventable-deaths.html.

2. Peter Suderman, "Bernie Sanders Thinks Medicare for All Could Cost $40 Trillion," *Reason*, July 17, 2019, https://reason.com/2019/07/17/bernie-sanders-medicare -for-all-cost-40-trillion-obamacare-single-payer/.

3. Amir Mirhaghi, Abbas Heydari, Mohsen Ebrahimi, et al. "Nonemergent Patients in the Emergency Department," *Trauma Monthly* 21, no. 4 (September 2016), doi: 10.5812/traumamon.23260.

4. bioMérieux, "Antibiotic-Resistant Infections Cost the U.S. Healthcare System in Excess of $20 Billion Annually," October 19, 2009, https://www.biomerieux-usa.com /antibiotic-resistant-infections-cost-us-healthcare-system-excess-20-billion-annually.

5. Centers for Disease Control and Prevention, "Untreatable: Report by CDC Details Today's Drug-Resistant Health Threats," September 16, 2013. https:// www.cdc.gov/media/releases/2013/p0916-untreatable.html.

6. Bruce Japsen, "Doctor Wait Times Soar 30% in Major U.S. Cities," *Forbes*, March 19, 2017, https://www.forbes.com/sites/brucejapsen/2017/03/19/doctor-wait -times-soar-amid-trumpcare-debate/#7ac4b5212e74.

7. Feixue Ren and Yanick Labrie, "Leaving Canada for Medical Care, 2017," *Fraser Research Bulletin* (June 2017), https://www.fraserinstitute.org/sites/default /files/leaving-canada-for-medical-care-2017.pdf.

8. "Doctors at Brink of Breaking Point to Ensure Patient Care, Warns Regulator," ITV, December 5, 2018, https://www.itv.com/news/2018-12-05/doctors-at-brink -of-breaking-point-to-ensure-patient-care-warns-regulator/.

9. Chris Smyth, "NHS Chiefs to Cut Host of Routine Operations," *The Times*, June 30, 2018, https://www.thetimes.co.uk/article/nhs-chiefs-to-cut-host-of-routine -operations-9k9sn3zpm.

10. Henry Bodkin, "Obese Patients and Smokers Banned from Routine Surgery in 'Most Severe Ever' Rationing in the NHS," *The Telegraph*, September 2, 2016, https://www.telegraph.co.uk/news/2016/09/02/obese-patients-and-smokers -banned-from-all-routine-operations-by/.

11. S. Sigurgeirsdóttir, J. Waagfjörð, and A. Maresso, "Iceland: Health System Review," *Health Systems in Transition* 16, no. 6 (2014): 1–182, https://www.ncbi.nlm.nih .gov/pubmed/25720021.

CHAPTER 10: THE AMERICAN HEALTH SYSTEM

1. Politifact, "Obama: 'If You Like Your Health Care Plan, You'll Be Able to Keep Your Health Care Plan,'"https://www.politifact.com/obama-like-health-care-keep/.
2. Jonah Goldberg, "Obama Health Lie Freaks Dems," *USA Today*, November 5, 2013, https://www.usatoday.com/story/opinion/2013/11/05/obama-health -care-lie-obamacare-column/3442423/.
3. Zirui Song, "Effect of a Workplace Wellness Program on Employee Health and Economic Outcomes," *JAMA* 321, no. 15 (2019): 1491–1501. doi:10.1001/jama .2019.3307.
4. Rebecca Greenfield, "Workplace Wellness Programmes Don't Work for You or Your Company, Study Finds," *Stuff*, January 28, 2018, https://www.stuff.co.nz /business/100959582/workplace-wellness-programmes-dont-work-for-you-or -your-company-study-finds.
5. "Market Value of Health and Wellness in the United States from 2015 to 2020 (in Million U.S. Dollars)," Statista, https://www.statista.com/statistics/491302 /health-and-wellness-united-states-market-value.
6. Julie Appleby, "How Well Do Workplace Wellness Programs Work?" NPR, April 16, 2019, https://www.npr.org/sections/health-shots/2019/04/16/713902890 /how-well-do-workplace-wellness-programs-work
7. Zirui Song, "Effect of a Workplace Wellness Program on Employee Health and Economic Outcomes," *JAMA* 321, no. 15 (2019): 1491–1501, doi:10.1001/jama .2019.3307.

CHAPTER 11: PERSONAL RESPONSIBILITY

1. Beth Baker, "Obesity's Hefty Price Tag," *Politico*, March 8, 2017, https://www .politico.com/agenda/story/2017/03/obesity-epidemic-in-america-healthcare -costs-000336; "Federal Spending: Where Does the Money Go," National Priorities Project, https://www.nationalpriorities.org/budget-basics/federal -budget-101/spending/.
2. Paul Bedard, "Obesity Epidemic at New High, Costs $150B a Year, Hurts Military Recruiting," *Washington Examiner*, September 1, 2017, https://www .washingtonexaminer.com/obesity-epidemic-at-new-high-costs-150b-a-year -hurts-military-recruiting.
3. "Where's the Sodium?" *CDC Vital Signs*, February 2012, https://www.cdc.gov /VitalSigns/pdf/2012-02-vitalsigns.pdf.
4. Marsha McCulloch, "30 Foods High in Sodium and What to Eat Instead," Healthline, September 9, 2018, https://www.healthline.com/nutrition/foods -high-in-sodium#section6.
5. "Excessive Drinking Is Draining the U.S. Economy," *CDC Features*, July 13, 2018, https://www.cdc.gov/features/costsofdrinking/index.html.
6. Aaron M. White, Megan Slater, Grace Ng, et. al, "Trends in Alcohol-Related

Emergency Department Visits in the United States," *Alcoholism: Clinical and Experimental Research*, 42, no. 2 (January 2, 2018), https://doi.org/10.1111/acer.13559.
7. Centers for Disease Control and Prevention, "Office on Smoking and Health at a Glance," May 25, 2009, https://www.cdc.gov/chronicdisease/resources/publications/aag/tobacco-use.htm.
8. Centers for Disease Control and Prevention, "Smoking Rates for Uninsured Adults on Medicaid More Than Twice Those for Adults with Private Health Insurance," press release, November 12, 2015, https://www.cdc.gov/media/releases/2015/p1112-smoking-rates.html.

ABOUT THE AUTHOR

NICOLE SAPHIER is a radiologist and breast cancer specialist at Memorial Sloan Kettering Cancer Center in New York City. She is frequently featured as a health policy expert and guest host on networks such as Fox News Channel and Fox Business Network. Dr. Saphier was awarded the Physician Champion Award for her efforts in passing multiple laws ensuring women have access to crucial cancer screening and treatment. She also plays an active part in her municipal, state, and federal legislative bodies. In addition to her professional roles, she is a mother to three boys and wife to a busy neurosurgeon living outside of New York City.